PREVENTIVE MEDICINE
USA

The John E. Fogarty International Center for Advanced Study in the Health Sciences

The Fogarty International Center was established in 1968 as a memorial to the late Congressman John E. Fogarty of Rhode Island. It had been Mr. Fogarty's desire to create within the National Institutes of Health a center for research in biology and medicine, dedicated to international cooperation and collaboration in the interest of the health of mankind. The Fogarty Center is a unique resource within the Federal establishment, providing a base for expanding of America's health research and health care to lands abroad and for bringing the talents and resources of other nations to bear upon the many and varied health problems of the United States.

As an institution for advanced study, the Center has embraced the major themes of medical education, environmental and societal factors influencing health, geographic health studies, preventive medicine, and biomedical research. The Center provides the opportunity for study and discussion of current issues in these and other fields by convening conferences and workshops which bring together U.S. and foreign scientists. In addition, the Center promotes the research of U.S. nationals at institutions abroad and the education and training of foreign scientists in the U.S. through a program of fellowships, scholarships, and study grants.

The American College of Preventive Medicine

The American College of Preventive Medicine is a professional society comprising physicians who are Board certified and/or engaged full time in preventive or community medicine. The membership includes individuals of scientific eminence in practice, teaching, or research in the specialty.

The College promotes continuing medical education and fosters interchange of knowledge and ideas among professionals in preventive medicine through annual meetings, conferences, publications, and joint activities with kindred professional societies.

The society was founded in 1954, six years after the establishment of the American Board of Preventive Medicine, the certifying specialty Board for physicians in the four preventive medicine subspecialties (Public Health, Aerospace Medicine, Occupational Medicine, and General Preventive Medicine).

As the only professional society whose membership encompasses all four subspecialties, the College provides a unique forum for physicians in preventive medicine to speak with one voice from an authoritative position to members of the government and organized medicine.

PREVENTIVE MEDICINE USA

Education and Training

of Health Manpower

for Prevention

A Task Force Report sponsored by

The John E. Fogarty International Center
for Advanced Study in the Health Sciences
National Institutes of Health

and

The American College of Preventive Medicine

PRODIST
New York
1976

Library of Congress Catalog Card Number 76-15084
International Standard Book Number 0-88202-106-0

PRODIST
a division of
Neale Watson Academic Publications, Inc.
156 Fifth Avenue, New York, New York 10010

Designed and manufactured in the U.S.A.

Contents

Preface

Improvement in the health status of the American people will depend, in great measure, on the design and application of programs which place major emphasis on the preventive aspects of human disease. The nature of our health problems dictates that application of known methodologies in prevention and health maintenance can cause a substantial improvement in our nation's health statistics. Although health authorities generally agree with this thesis, there is need for more precise definition of effective methods and programs of prevention, financial and manpower resources required to implement these programs, and priorities to be assigned to research in preventive methodology.

Leaders throughout the health field, in government, the academic sector, and industry, have expressed repeatedly the need to assemble expertise in order to elucidate mechanisms whereby the full impact of preventive medicine can be brought to bear on the solution of America's major health problems. The Department of Health, Education, and Welfare has evidenced its commitment to prevention in a variety of ways, the most notable being that prevention has been selected as one of the five major themes for development in Departmental programs, as detailed in *The Forward Plan for Health, 1976-1980.* As stated there, "the major element of a preventive strategy is to assure the concentration of all federally supported health programs in preventive health services, health maintenance, and health education." The Department has pledged a full commitment to review of current practice, evaluation of preventive methodology, and the generation of new knowledge.

The Fogarty International Center of the National Institutes of Health, in anticipation of this new emphasis, initiated in 1973 an analysis of preventive medicine. Comprehensive studies were designed to review and evaluate the state-of-the-art of prevention and control of human diseases, to identify deficiencies in knowledge requiring further research, and to recognize problems in application of preventive methods and suggest corrective action. In an effort to contribute to the educational aspects of preventive medicine, the Fogarty Center undertook a cooperative program with the Association of Teachers of Preventive Medicine to conduct workshops and create resource material to assist in the administration, teaching, research, and service responsibilities of departments of preventive medicine, to enhance collaborative activities between these departments and other units of health science schools, and to promote national programs of teaching, research, and service in preventive medicine.

These efforts in preventive medicine, and the close collaboration with experts in this and allied fields, led the Fogarty Center and the American

College of Preventive Medicine to create and support the work of eight Task Forces addressing various components of the field of disease prevention, whose charge was to develop guidelines for a national effort in preventive medicine. The output was to be specifics; that is, concrete proposals whose orientations were pragmatic, programmatic, and realistic. Over 300 specialists participated in preparing these documents with the endorsement and support of health organizations and professional societies with preventive medicine orientations. In June, 1975, the eight reports were presented at the National Conference on Preventive Medicine convened at the National Institutes of Health. The major purposes of the conference were to focus attention on the significant accomplishments of preventive strategies that had been applied to the health problems of this country in recent years and to offer expert opinion on where preventive measures could be expected to yield equally significant health advances in the future. At this meeting, the reports were analyzed during workshop sessions, and their recommendations were discussed and revised until a scientific consensus was reached. The present volume is the culmination of this concerned, long-term effort.

The eight Task Force reports were used as the basis for the Prevention theme of the DHEW *Forward Plan for Health, 1976-1980*, and the recommendations of the reports are being considered by DHEW agency heads for appropriate implementation in their programs. While the debate will continue as to the precise Federal role in developing and executing a national health plan, most observers recognize the paramount position of the Congress and the Executive branch in formulating guidelines for system reform. We anticipate that the documents of the National Conference on Preventive Medicine will provide a base of knowledge on the theory and application of preventive medicine from which national programs might arise.

Milo D. Leavitt, Jr., M.D.
Director
Fogarty International Center

Irving Tabershaw, M.D.
President
American College of Preventive Medicine

Task Force Members

John H. Bryant, M.D., *Chairman*
Director
School of Public Health
Columbia University
New York, New York

Ramona E. F. Arnett, A.B.
Administrative Director
Center for Educational
  Development in Health
School of Public Health
Harvard University
Boston, Massachusetts

William H. Barker, Jr., M.D.
Medical Officer
Office of Program Planning
  and Evaluation
Center for Disease Control
Atlanta, Georgia

Thornton Bryan, M.D.
Professor and Chairman
Department of Family Medicine
College of Medicine
The University of Tennessee
Memphis, Tennessee

Noreen M. Clark, M.A.
Director, Program of
  Continuing Education, and
Assistant Professor,
  Health Administration
School of Public Health
Columbia University
New York, New York

John Colombotos, PH.D.
Associate Professor of
  Sociomedical Sciences
School of Public Health
Columbia University
New York, New York

Jere E. Goyan, PH.D.
Dean
School of Pharmacy
University of California
San Francisco, California

Thomas L. Hall, M.D.
Acting Director
Carolina Population Center
University of North Carolina
Chapel Hill, North Carolina

Thelma Ingles, M.A., R.N.
Visiting Professor of Research
School of Nursing
University of North Carolina
Chapel Hill, North Carolina

Rudolph E. Micik, D.D.S., M.S.
Educational Specialist
Education Development Branch
Division of Dentistry
Bureau of Health Resources
  Development
Health Resources Administration
Bethesda, Maryland

Max Pepper, M.D.
Professor and Chairman
Department of Community Medicine
School of Medicine
St. Louis University
St. Louis, Missouri

1

J. Warren Perry, PH.D.
Dean
School of Health Related
  Professions
State University of New York
Buffalo, New York

William P. Richardson, M.D.
Professor of Preventive Medicine
Department of Family Medicine
School of Medicine
University of North Carolina
Chapel Hill, North Carolina

Mitchell Schorow, PH.D.
Coordinator for
  Educational Development
College of Physicians
  and Surgeons
Columbia University
New York, New York

Raymond Seltser, M.D., M.P.H.
Associate Dean
School of Hygiene and
  Public Health
The Johns Hopkins University
Baltimore, Maryland

Reuel A. Stallones, M.D., M.P.H.
Dean
School of Public Health
University of Texas
Houston, Texas

Michael M. Stewart, M.D.
Director
Department of Ambulatory Care
  and Community Medicine
Mount Sinai Hospital Services
City Hospital Center at Elmhurst
Elmhurst, New York

Irving R. Tabershaw, M.D.
President
Tabershaw-Cooper Associates, Inc.
Rockville, Maryland

Ina Tranberg
President
Local 1251
District Council 37
American Federation of State,
  County and Municipal Employees
New York, New York

Introduction

This report draws on the collective expertise and thoughtful participation of all of the members of this Task Force. Virtually every person has made a substantive contribution to its content—by writing, by reviewing what was written, or, not least of all, simply by raising thoughtful questions and challenging glib assumptions during our meetings.

Some of the individual papers contained herein are signed by those Task Force members who prepared them. Those individual authors wish it to be understood that the opinions set forth in their signed pieces are their own and do not necessarily represent the official views of any organizations with which they are affiliated. The unsigned pieces represent a collaborative effort of Task Force V members.

It would have been virtually impossible for any single one of us to have generalized about educational and training needs for prevention without interjecting a personal bias or a particular professional focus. Since the document reflects so many points of view, it is probably a more useful and true-to-life assessment of what changes in professional education would be required to launch a truly comprehensive and effective national preventive endeavor than any individual or small-group effort could have been. We hope it will be helpful to those concerned with the future of preventive health care in the United States.

The basic assumption that underlies our examination of education and training of health personnel is that no matter what the content of curricula is or how much emphasis is put on preventive services in training programs for health personnel, truly effective and comprehensive health care will not become a reality unless there is a corresponding change in institutional and national policy toward prevention. One of the things that all providers must learn if they are to be effective (they may not be *taught* it in a classroom, but they learn it nonetheless) is how to work within—or, at any rate, around—the system; nothing, therefore, will really change at the bottom unless the system also changes at the top.

On the other hand, any change in policy toward the provision of preventive services will have little effect unless it also takes into account the changes in academic curricula and training programs, and in the research-derived knowledge base that underlies those programs, that will be needed to produce providers with a preventive orientation. Health care policy makers can mandate all the preventive services that they can think of, but if health workers are neither equipped nor inclined to provide such services, prevention will not occur.

(To avoid confusion, the term "prevention" or "preventive health care," rather than "preventive medicine," will be used throughout this

3

report to refer to those preventive interventions that are not exclusively in the domain of the physician specialist in preventive medicine. The term "preventive medicine" will be reserved throughout for the specialty itself.)

What goes on in the classroom or training site can have a significant effect upon health care policy and organization; at the same time, however, the system dictates the kind of training that will be best and most frequently rewarded—by money, prestige, and provider satisfaction. Keeping this rather paradoxical symbiotic situation well in mind, Task Force V identified its challenge in terms of the following series of questions:

1. Who should have responsibility for prevention? (Our assumption from the outset was that all health personnel and the public would be eligible for consideration.)
2. What are the health care settings in which preventive concepts can be implemented?
3. What are the roles of physicians in prevention, and what is the specific role of specialists in preventive medicine?
4. What is the current state of education and training for preventive health care?
5. What should be the content of educational and training programs for prevention?
6. What methods should be used in educating and training health personnel for prevention?
7. What should the interrelationships be among education and training programs in prevention for different categories of health manpower?
8. What is the role of continuing education in preventive health care?
9. What aspects of education and training for prevention require further research?
10. What amounts and channels of funding are required to develop and maintain education and training for prevention at desirable levels?

This list was a starting point for our deliberations. Recognizing, however, that not all of these areas could be considered in detail, we determined that we should take an empirical approach of (1) definition, (2) analysis, and (3) synthesis and solution. The present form of this report roughly corresponds to those divisions, with Parts II and III both being analytical.

We tried to start with as few assumptions as possible in order to gain new insights into our subject and avoid as much as possible falling back on pat, rhetorical statements about the inadequacies of educational and training systems. We did, however, have to make a few basic initial assumptions, to wit, what the objectives of prevention should be and what

4

the practice of prevention should entail, in order to have a base from which to analyze the educational and training components, both actual and ideal, of that practice. Part I of this document reports on some of our efforts to arrive at a definition of prevention in health care that would be commonly understood—if not always completely agreed upon—by the members of this Task Force.

Parts II and III of this report, our analysis of the state of the art, essentially consist of a series of working papers that utilize several diagnostic approaches in order to expose the more obvious discrepancies between the way preventive health care is presently taught—or, as is often the case, *not* taught—and the educational and training needs in this area. The "tracer" analyses of selected categories of health personnel (some of which are included in the text and the rest of which can be found in Appendix A), along with the corresponding quantitative analyses of manpower needs for prevention, were very helpful in highlighting some of these discrepancies.

Part II deals with a wife range of health personnel, while Part III concentrates specifically on physician specialists in preventive medicine. Although these two parts of the report and the documents included in Appendix A by no means constitute a comprehensive survey, we did find that there were features common to all of the manpower categories considered from which we could generalize. Although the Task Force's specific recommendations based on these findings will be set forth in Part IV of this report, it is perhaps appropriate to consider briefly here the generalizations derived from our analyses in the wider context of the health care system at large.

From the Task Force discussions and working documents emerged a large number of issues that seemed to cluster into the five areas listed below, which serve as the focal points for the conclusions and suggestions made in Part IV. They begin with the premise that there should be, and indeed will be, a national program of prevention, and proceed to address the following implications for education and training if such a national effort is to be effective.

1. *The knowledge base for preventive health care.* Preventive programs are heavily dependent on the knowledge base derived through basic research and field studies and on the dissemination of this knowledge through education and training. Continued and increased support of research and research training is an essential ingredient for an effective national program of preventive health care.

2. *The preventive content in education and training.* Existing educational and training programs for health personnel are often seriously deficient in preventive components. These deficiencies are due to lack of attention to prevention by legislators, educators, and providers, and

5

thereby to inadequacies in funding, program design, and what might be called educational enthusiasm. Major changes are called for both in the support given and requirements mandated by legislation and in the aggressiveness and innovativeness with which educational institutions approach this important area.

3. *The management of the learning setting for prevention.* Substantial challenges and opportunities lie in the ways in which education and training programs can be structured in educational institutions and in the linkages they can have with operational programs in the health care system. At stake are issues such as interdisciplinary education, avoiding duplication in health sciences centers of educational resources for prevention, and the relevance of educational programs to operational practicalities of health care.

4. *The educational and training continuum.* The discontinuities, fragmentation, and plain lack of opportunities that characterize current approaches to continuing education and training present serious obstacles to mounting an effective national program of prevention. There is a need to develop as a planned continuum alternative approaches for providing opportunities for career-long education and training, including programs for professional upgrading, preparation for certification and recertification, and mechanisms for making mid-career professional changes.

5. *Health manpower needs for prevention.* While the argument can be made for planning for health manpower development on a rational quantitative basis, it is clear that the data base for such planning is seriously inadequate. Data systems for manpower planning must therefore receive immediate attention, together with research-based approaches to manpower planning. At the same time, however, available information is sufficient to justify taking early steps to increase the supply of certain manpower categories that are critical to a preventive effort.

Looking across these challenges, it is apparent that many of the deficiencies and obstacles to education and training for prevention lie in a lack of interest, knowledge, and commitment to prevention as an important and cost-effective part of health care. While the Congress (in the National Health Planning and Development Act) and the Department of Health, Education, and Welfare (in its Forward Plan for 1975–1980) have been unequivocal in placing prevention among the top priorities of future health care development, actual progress in making comprehensive preventive health care a reality will require supportive action on a number of fronts, of which education and training is an essential one. There must be a heightened awareness among educational institutions, faculties, professional societies, and legislators of the areas of preventive intervention that are practical and effective and of developments relative to education and training that are essential to support a national effort in prevention.

6

Part I: Scope of Personnel, Settings, and Services for Prevention

Before undertaking any substantive analysis of the present state of education for prevention, much less making recommendations for what can and should be done in this area, this Task Force found it necessary to formulate a working definition of what preventive health care is and who may provide it. As a handle to permit us at least to begin discussion, we initially accepted the definition of the American College of Preventive Medicine (ACPM), which we paraphrased thus:

> The primary focus of preventive medicine is health and disease as these occur in communities and in defined population groups. Preventive medicine seeks to promote those practices with respect to the community and the individual that will advance health, prevent disease, make possible early diagnosis and treatment, and foster rehabilitation of those with disabilities.

When, in the light of this definition, we considered (1) who should be responsible for prevention, (2) in what settings preventive intervention could occur, and (3) what kinds of activities constitute preventive health care, we came to the following conclusions:

1. *Who should be responsible for prevention?* All categories of health manpower, plus policy makers and the public, are involved in prevention in its broadest sense. Thus the Task Force decided that its focus should not be primarily on specialists in preventive medicine, nor even mainly on physicians. We concluded that, at the very least, we should consider the following categories of health workers:

A. Physician specialists in preventive medicine: clinical, nonclinical (administration, research, education, etc.);

B. Primary care physicians: internists, pediatricians, obstetrician-gynecologists, family physicians, general practitioners;

C. Other physician specialists: clinical and nonclinical;

D. Physician extenders: physician's assistants, nurse-practitioners (family nurse-practitioners, pediatric nurse-practitioners, nurse-midwives, etc.), MEDEX;

(We recognize that in many settings the nurse-practitioner functions as an essentially autonomous provider of care and should in those circumstances be considered as a separate category of manpower rather than as physician extenders.)

E. Nurses and nurse auxiliaries: registered nurses, public health nurses, clinical specialists, nurse epidemiologists, etc.; licensed practical nurses, nurse's aides, etc.;

F. Dentists and dental auxiliaries: "typical" office-based generalists; dental hygienists, dental assistants, etc.;
G. Pharmacists ("typical" practicing pharmacists) and pharmaceutical assistants;
H. Mental health workers;
I. Allied health workers: occupational health workers; physical therapists; nutritionists, dieticians; etc.;
J. Social workers;
K. Sanitarians and environmentalists: FDA inspectors; public health advisors;
L. Managers of health care institutions;
M. Individual consumers.

(We were unable in the scope of our examination to devote time to the concept of self-care; we wish, however, to acknowledge our opinion that this is an area that any truly comprehensive national policy on preventive health care should take into consideration.)

Although we were unanimous in our feeling that prevention is not, nor should it be, the exclusive property of the specialist in preventive medicine, we recognized that there are certain specialized aspects relating to prevention, most clearly definable in terms of the community approach to community health problems, that are primarily the province of physicians who concentrate on prevention as their medical specialty and chief professional interest. We also recognized that specialists in preventive medicine are the most likely candidates for broadening the base of knowledge in prevention and for teaching preventive activities to other health care professionals. For all of these reasons, therefore—and in accordance with our mandate—we have devoted a portion of our deliberations and an entire part of this report (see Part III) to a consideration of the educational and training components of the specialty of preventive medicine.

2. *In what settings can preventive intervention occur?* If we followed the ACPM definition, it was clear that prevention—in the broadest sense of the word—could occur in a great variety of settings, including at least all of the following and probably many others as well:

A. Federal agencies (Center for Disease Control, Food and Drug Administration);
B. Hospitals (community hospitals, referral hospitals, specialty hospitals);
C. State and local health departments;
D. Health centers/satellite clinics;
E. Private offices (solo or group practices);
F. Mobile units (screening programs);

8

G. Schools;

H. Place of work (offices, factories, institutions);

I. Place of leisure activity (clubs, community centers, etc.);

J. Home.

3. *What kinds of activities constitute preventive health care?* According to the ACPM definition, the scope of prevention includes health promotion, disease prevention, early diagnosis and treatment, and rehabilitation—in other words, primary, secondary, and tertiary prevention. We found that the schematic diagram of the health care system in Fig. 1 was helpful in pinpointing the stages at which these levels of preventive intervention can occur.

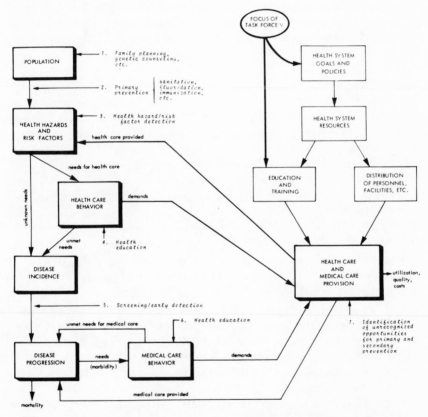

Source: Adapted from Richard D. Smallwood, "A Quantitative Approach to Analyzing Regional Health Care Systems", Program in Health Care System Analysis, Stanford University, 1971 (mimeograph).

Fig. 1. Structural Model for Points of Preventive Intervention in the Health Care System

9

Having come this far in trying to define the scope of preventive health care, we found, however, that we were not much closer than when we started to having a manageable subject with which to work. The general feeling of the Task Force was that if we were to get on with our job, we should narrow our focus somewhat. It was suggested and agreed that we concentrate our attention on education und training principally for primary and certain aspects of secondary prevention, since, beyond those areas, preventive health care overlaps with clinical medical care and rehabilitative medicine.

Part II. Diagnostic Approaches for Determining Educational and Training Needs for Prevention

In Task Force V's attempts to be as systematic and representative (since we could not be comprehensive) as possible in our examination of the educational training needs for various kinds of health personnel, we hit upon several diagnostic approaches that helped us immeasurably in directing and developing our thinking. One of these diagnostic tools—a three-dimensional *matrix* of the preventive health care system, showing (1) providers of preventive services, (2) preventive activities, and (3) the target populations for preventive intervention on the three axes—became the starting point for another method we used in our analysis of the state of the art, a *tracer* technique for identifying the preventive roles and corresponding educational needs of a variety of health manpower. Using this tracer approach for analyzing the functions, and the educational preparation for those functions, of different categories of preventive health care workers permitted us to assess better who is doing what and where in prevention and, by extension, what is wrong with basic professional education, continuing education, field placement, and style of work. The tracer analyses of individual providers that are included in this report each conclude with a section on the quantification of those categories of manpower, adding another important dimension to our investigation of the "who, what, and for whom?" of prevention—the "how many?"

Having dealt in passing with such influences on the practice of prevention as training, financing, and the organization of the health care system, Part II concludes with an examination of another factor that determines to a considerable degree the extent to which prevention is practiced, that being the provider's *attitudes* toward preventive health care.

The Prevention Matrix

Using the three-dimensional matrix shown on in Fig. 2, we addressed the following questions:

1. What major preventive activities are these, or any other, categories of health workers involved in? ("Involved" could be interpreted as meaning active in planning, supervision, direct participation, sustained advocacy, etc.)
2. What cells of the matrix reflect the bulk of these activities?
3. How adequate and appropriate are these activities?

11

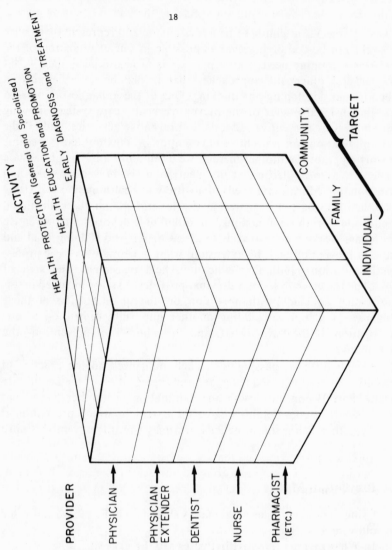

Fig. 2. The Prevention Matrix

4. What are the implications for education and training of these categories of health workers to perform these preventive interventions?

If one "asked" the matrix many questions about which health workers provide what preventive services for what target groups, one would, no doubt, end up with some cells of the matrix showing a great deal of activity and others showing relatively little; thus the matrix does have the potential for giving us a diagnostic view of what the current state of affairs is in regard to prevention. Like any such simple schematic approach to a complicated problem, however, the matrix has its limitations. Not only does it in no way reflect a qualitative judgment of current preventive activity, but also, and obviously, where the weight presently is and where it should be are two different matters—i.e., it only demonstrates what we think *is* happening (which is arbitrary to begin with); it does not show who *should* be doing what and where.

One of the manpower tracer analyses that follows, that for the pharmacist, attempts to overcome this drawback by using two matrices to illustrate the pharmacist's preventive role, one representing his *actual* current functions, the other showing his *potential* activities in prevention.

The labels on the axes of the matrix can be changed to give a diagnostic view of whatever aspect of preventive health care one wishes to examine. It can be used to analyze the functions of any given kind of health worker by including only that single provider on the provider axis; to examine the various services provided by a certain category of professionals (e.g., general dentist, periodontist, orthodontist, etc.); or to compare the functions of different types of health personnel working in the same field (e.g., obstetrician, nurse-midwife, obstetrical nurse). The target axis could likewise be changed. For example, in the examination in this report of the role of the physician specialist in occupational medicine, a fourth target, industry, turned out to be a logical addition to the three shown in the matrix illustrated here.

Although no meaningful conclusions can be drawn from the matrices themselves, they did have value for Task Force V by helping us to focus our thinking better. We found that they were a useful starting point in our examination of the preventive roles of the selected categories of manpower that constitute the tracer analyses on the following pages and in Appendix A of this report.

Selected Categories of Health Personnel as Tracers for the Practice of Prevention

Methodology

The outline below shows the steps used in the following sections to trace the roles and functions of the categories of health workers consid-

13

ered and to identify implications for the education of these professionals. An attempt was made to determine the discrepancies between current practice and the desired level of professional performance in the following manner:

1. The previously discussed provider/activity/target matrix was used to identify the major activity areas for which the type of health worker under consideration has responsibility and the populations for which preventive services are provided.

2. The responsibilities and functions of any given category of provider as identified by its respective professional associations were considered vis-a-vis the issues and concerns in prevention that were identified by Task Force V. A listing of those areas in which current practice appears effective was compiled. This list indicates the *adequacies* of that group of health personnel. A listing of discrepancies between current and desired practice was compiled. This represents the *inadequacies* of these health workers.

3. The listing of inadequacies was examined for contributing factors. Each factor was related to specific aspects of the health system:

| policy | financing | interrelationships |
| structure | education | |

4. These inadequacies and the factors contributing to them were analyzed to identify educational principles and relationships that would lead to improved professional practice.

This outline was adopted, with individual modifications, by various members of Task Force V to identify the discrepancies between the actual and the ideal practice of prevention by a wide range of health care providers. In all, seven such tracers were prepared, three of which follow here, one of which is included in Part III, and the remainder of which can be found in Appendix A of this report. The selection of the categories of personnel for tracer analysis was a purely arbitrary one, based more on the personal interests and the firsthand knowledge of those Task Force members who prepared the tracers than on any attempt to be systematic or comprehensive in our analysis. Not all of the tracers follow exactly the outline given above. Because they were prepared by individual members of Task Force V, they have individual variations—some are descriptive, and others are problem-oriented; some are rather idealized, others quite realistic.

Despite these individual differences in approach, however, and despite the fact that the seven types of manpower considered constitute only a very small proportion of the numbers and kinds of health personnel that have (or should have) responsibility for prevention, what emerges from these tracers is fairly panoramic view of how preventive services are currently provided and how they might better be. Taken together, the recommendations set forth in each tracer for improving the preventive component of the education and training that each category of health personnel receives (corresponding to #4 in the tracer outline above) point to some of the interdisciplinary guidelines and recommendations given in Part IV of this report.

Each of the tracers concludes with a section on the *quantification* of that category of manpower for prevention. The greater part of this report is devoted to the *qualitative* aspects of health manpower training in preventive medicine—who needs training, for what reasons, what kind of training, and how adequate the current training programs are at the undergraduate, specialty, and refresher training levels. These quantitative sections, therefore, seek to provide a rough numerical dimension to some of these questions. This objective is important, for without quantification, policy makers and educators will have little basis upon which to establish training targets and to allocate resources. At the same time it is fraught with at least three major methodological perils: (1) Of all health personnel who should have training for prevention, only a small proportion are specialists in this field and have clearly defined programs in the subject; (2) available data for most training programs are not sufficiently detailed to allow judgments to be made regarding the adequacy of the preventive component or even to allow estimation of the potential training capacity of programs; and (3) reliable supply information is hardly adequate even for the preventive medicine specialist, much less for the many manpower categories where preventive health care represents an important but not dominant part of their training. For this last-named category there is no easy way of distinguishing between those with adequate training and those who should receive supplementary or refresher training, nor for converting the number needing supplementary training in prevention into the number who would actually seek such training if it were readily available.

Given these and other important constraints to the quantification of training needs, it seemed prudent to limit our inquiries pretty much to those manpower categories that are analyzed by the tracer method. These categories are used by way of illustrating both the possible magnitude of the training task (not only how many health workers need to be trained in prevention, but also, by inference, how many *teachers* will be needed for the task, which has specific implications for the quantification of preventive medicine specialists), as well as possible approaches to deriving such estimates. The assumptions used in each case are identified, and where the reader has reason to prefer different assumptions, he is invited to test their implications on the resultant projections of training needs.

Looking beyond the few individual manpower categories considered here and taking instead a collective look at the entire health manpower

15

pool, one realizes that there is a heartening supply of people who can each contribute in some way to preventive endeavors. The challenge for policy makers and educators alike is to find ways of both maximizing the potential of the existing supply and increasing the supply in those categories in which more manpower for prevention is critically needed.

Tracer: Community Health Education Specialist

This tracer was prepared by Noreen M. Clark, M.A., with the assistance of Irving Shapiro, PH.D., Adjunct Associate Professor, Columbia University School of Public Health, and Anna F. Skiff, M.P.H., Education Officer, United States Public Health Service Hospital, Staten Island, N.Y.

Role. In order to place the community health education specialist in the prevention matrix, it is necessary to look at the role of education in health promotion and maintenance. Participation in education is believed to contribute to an individual's ability to think creatively, solve problems intelligently, and achieve self-reliance. Health education is a way to give individuals a broader base for responsible decisionmaking and to assist them in engaging in actions that promote, maintain, or restore their own health.

The Report of the Task Force on Consumer Health Education of the National Conference on Preventive Medicine points out that the term frequently used by persons in this field is "professional health educator"— presumably to distinguish them from everyone else engaged in health education. The term is misleading in that it implies that other health professions involved in health education are not professionally trained. The alternative phrase "health education specialist" is thus used in that report and will be used here also.

The health educator has historically been the health professional who has viewed humans and their health more holistically than others. If we recognize that human beings are where they are on the health/disease continuum because of an interplay of biological, physical, social, and cultural factors, then we must recognize that education for prevention and health promotion cannot be reductionistic or atomistic. As John Hanlon points out, taking an ecological perspective "forces us to look at the whole human organism not just its organs and organ system, much less in terms of interests of particular professions. It forces us to view the environment as being, in reality, multi-environments integrated into a remarkable system."[1]

The health educator draws from the biological, physical, behavioral, and social sciences a mass of knowledge and skills to be applied in a variety of settings and at many intervention points. Other health workers

16

also have educational responsibilities, but it is the health educator who has particular knowledge of what educational principles are appropriate at which time and place. Education is clearly a primary aspect of any program in prevention. The health educator is the specially trained individual who is continually and consistently aware of and responsible for optimizing the educational component. He or she both plans and implements educational programs and helps other health workers develop their educational capacity.

Health education contributes to prevention and health promotion by helping individuals, through the educator's appreciation of the social, psychological, and cultural influences on their behavior, develop an understanding of and appropriate reactions to health, disease, and living, and by delineating, testing, and refining educational concepts and practices that contribute to better health behavior.

Functions. Given the above, it is apparent that all aspects of the health educator's practice relate to prevention, and his/her areas of responsibility correspond, at least indirectly, to virtually all cells of the activity/target matrix.

The community health educator is prepared to assume a wide range of functions, many of which are rarely carried out by others. The functions outlined are adapted from the "Statement of Functions of Community Health Educators," which was adopted by the Board of the Society of Public Health Education in March 1967. In assuming these functions, the educator employs a variety of methods and techniques to reach the goal of assisting individuals and communities to promote, maintain, and restore their own health. Some of the strengths in health education practice are:

1. identifying community resources and structure of community leadership;
2. establishing and maintaining lines of communication with community organizations and agencies;
3. identifying those health issues determined to be priorities in the community;
4. developing educational programs, methods, and materials;
5. training staff; and
6. coordinating and acting as liaison with health agencies and organizations.

There are other functions and responsibilities health educators are expected to carry out that, for many reasons (some of which will be mentioned later), may be especially difficult to achieve. Among these inadequacies in practice are:

1. helping the agencies who employ them to formulate policy related

17

to individual and community health education and health promotion;

2. understanding the complexities of disease processes and the appropriate preventive measures (what is effective, when, and for whom);

3. assessing specific learning needs of individuals and communities related to both personal health and participation in the health system;

4. engaging in collaboration with individuals and communities to establish shared goals;

5. identifying specific and measurable objectives and designing techniques and procedures to determine whether they have been met;

6. educating individuals and communities for responsibility in promoting, maintaining, and restoring their own health; and

7. obtaining funds for education in prevention and health promotion.

Obstacles to Practice. In order for community health education specialists to function optimally they must first of all be prepared through professional training and, secondly, work in a setting where it is possible to carry out the functions for which they have been prepared. Hindrances to effective practice may therefore arise from many factors, including policies related to health education, prevention, and health promotion; the existing health system structure and relationships; existing arrangements for financing health education; and the education of community health education practitioners. For example:

1. Policy: It is difficult for a community health educator to influence his/her agency or institution in favor of prevention and health promotion if these are not priorities of the health field in general.

2. Structure: The community health education specialist may not be included in decisionmaking at the appropriate level within the institution or agency to assure effective programming.

There may be a general lack of knowledge about health education, especially among those with primary patient responsibilities, resulting in education being given low priority as a component of health care or programs in prevention.

Health education programs may not be closely enough connected to the constituencies they aim to serve.

The community health education specialist may be isolated from or located at the periphery of the major health care and prevention activities in an institution or facility.

3. Interrelationships: Health education practice may be inhibited by the apparent cultural bias against teachers in our society, as demonstrated

by their relatively low pay, low prestige, and a prevailing sentiment that anyone can teach as well as anyone else.

The community health educator may not be viewed by those with primary patient responsibility as an equal member of the health care team; health education may therefore be compromised by lack of shared responsibility for decisionmaking, planning, etc.

The community health educator is concerned with the education both of individuals and the community and of other health professionals. This means the health educator must be accepted on two levels.

4. Financing: The role the community health educator is able to play has been conditioned by the profit-oriented nature of our society. Money allocated to employ health educators has often supported this marketplace view. Many medical service organizations either have severe budget limitations or conceptualize their operations solely in terms of cost/benefit. Consequently, they either have not hired educators at all or, where they have, have distorted their role, frequently requiring the educator to function as a public relations person or a fund-raiser.

The lack of appropriate levels and measures for funding or reimbursement of health education programs results in insufficient numbers of activities and/or insufficient impact.

There are many critical aspects of health care and prevention which cannot be computed in terms of cost alone. Although more evaluative data are needed, administrators and health systems managers who continue to view health education as contingent on traditional cost/benefit analysis hinder the establishment of programs.

5. Education: The supply of trained community health educators is small relative to the wide range of intervention points where education is an important component.[2]

Because the quality of the training of such people has been variable, not all health educators develop all the concepts and skills necessary to perform effectively. Thus the already small pool of qualified health educators is reduced still further, pointing to a greater need for appropriate training of a greater number of health educators.

Implications for Education and Training in Prevention and Health Promotion. Given these issues and the broad role the community health educator assumes in prevention and health promotion, some principles and relationships emerge that need to be emphasized in respect to the education and training of community health education specialists. Many of these points are contained in the "Criteria and Guidelines for Accrediting Graduate Programs in Community Health Education," Committee on Professional Education, *American Journal of Public Health, 59,* no. 3 (March 1969), and "Statement of Functions of Community Health Educators and Minimum Requirements for their Professional Preparation," Society for Public Health Education, March 1967. Each point presented here is of particular importance to efforts in prevention and health promotion.

1. Programs for educating the community health education specialist must continue to reintegrate concepts and skills from the behavioral and physical sciences in order to produce professionals with a holistic view of people and their health.

2. Educational programs for health educators need operational links; that is, they need to be associated with agencies that actually engage in education for prevention and health promotion. These agencies should comprise an appropriate spectrum of settings that reflect the wide variety of possible educational interventions. In addition, what the health educator needs to learn should be evident from the settings in which he/she is trained.

3. Education about the complexities of disease processes and the application of specific preventive measures is necessary in the preparation of community health educators. The health educator needs to learn problem-solving techniques that can be utilized in a great variety of situations; the issues of prevention and the complexities of disease lend themselves well to a problem-oriented approach.

4. The health educator must learn the appropriate levels and leverage points for influencing institutional decision and policy making.

5. Researchers in educational systems can contribute to the practice of health education by broadening its scientific base.[3] Interdisciplinary research is needed on how a variety of factors interact to influence particular behaviors or states of health. Much health behavior research is reductionistic and the value of its applicability misjudged. In order to address needs in health education practice, research must contribute to the *merging* of disciplines, not just to isolated aspects of health and disease.

6. Community assessment by the health educator to determine learning needs is essential to effective health education. Practical, intuitive, on-the-job assessment often may be the most effective means of determining these needs. This underscores the need for health educators to be directly involved with their prospective clients (communities, individuals, groups, organizations) during the period of academic training to learn community dynamics and educational assessment.

7. It is necessary for community health education specialists to be knowledgeable in the techniques and procedures of evaluation, in order to document success in reaching educational objectives. Expertise should also be developed in cost/benefit evaluation. According to Lawrence Green, "although it may be unfortunate that health education, which deals with humanitarian and philosophical goals, must be defended on

20

economic grounds, it appears that this is necessary if health education is to survive."[4]

8. If a goal of education is to assist individuals, families, and communities in assuming responsibility for their own health, health educators must be trained in programs that reflect this concept. This implies that the structure for training educators must include principles of individual responsibility, collaboration for shared objectives, emphasis on individual initiative, etc. The assumption—and a valid one, we feel—is that health educators who are trained according to such principles will teach as they were taught.

9. Development of education and training in health education will depend on the extent to which it is a priority of the health field. This involves and in fact depends on providing incentives through allocation of dollars for education, health promotion, and prevention. This need for incentives is emphasized in the report of a recent federal conference on health education:

> The long neglect in support of health education has created overwhelming need for manpower development. In addition, the present high expectations for the contribution health education can make to the solution of health problems and the enhancement of the general well-being of the population is creating an increased demand for service. Therefore inservice education and mid-career training of many existing practitioners are required, as well as the preparation of a large cadre of well-trained health education workers at all levels.[5]

Manpower Considerations. This section of the tracer was written by Thomas L. Hall, M.D., who, in collaboration with the individual tracer authors, supplied a quantitative analysis of manpower needs for all of the tracers included in this report.

The health education specialist is clearly a manpower category whose effectiveness depends in large part on an intimate knowledge of the concepts and applications of preventive medicine. The roles and functions of this health profession are described in still greater detail than above in the *Report of the Task Force on Consumer Health Education,* where a review of available supply and requirements estimates is also included.

The Report of the President's Committee on Health Education cited that in 1972 there were 25,000 professional health educators in school and community health education.[6] Dr. Scott Simonds, in a document prepared for the Task Force on Consumer Health Education, disagrees strongly with that estimate.[7] Simonds reviewed the recent literature on health education manpower, and the paragraphs that follow are taken largely from his report.

Present Supply. Rosemary Kent has estimated the current supply of personnel trained in schools of public health or other American Public Health Association (APHA)-accredited programs in community health education at the master's level and beyond and who are employed in public health education work as something under 1,100.[8] Attrition, for whatever reason, is accounted for in this estimate. Another estimate is 2,000 to 3,000,[9] a figure cited as having been provided by the Society for Public Health Education. This latter estimate probably takes into account personnel trained in health education at the master's level or beyond from other institutions as well as schools of public health and APHA-accredited programs.

An ad hoc Task Force on Professional Health Manpower for Community Health Programs that was convened in 1973 estimates the current supply of employed public health educators at 2,000.[10] That task force based its projection on the estimate of 1,800 health educators having graduated from accredited master's-level programs up to 1970.[11]

Estimates on currently available personnel trained at the bachelor's level or beyond with a major specialization in health education in a setting other than a school of public health are virtually nonexistent. Most persons trained in such programs enter school health education work. An estimate of the number of school health educators employed in 1971 was 20,000,[12] but the statistic is not documented and likely includes persons employed in school health education who have not been specifically prepared for that field. The American Alliance for Health, Physical Education, and Recreation has reported approximately 4,000 members as citing school health education as their primary field,[13] out of a total organizational membership of around 30,000.

The American School Health Association reported 8,000 members who were school health educators in 1971,[14] but similarly this group also includes personnel trained in nursing and other disciplines.

The figure of 25,000 professionally trained health educators cited earlier is a "guesstimate" at best and is based on organizational memberships perhaps more than anything else.

In all likelihood, a better estimate of the total number of individuals prepared in health education at the baccalaureate, master's, or doctoral levels and working actively in the field of either public health education or school health education would be no more than 12,500, and those prepared in community or public health education would account for no more than 2,000 of this total.[15] In any case, it is clear that a more definitivᴀ study of health education manpower is needed than has been done.

Projected Supply. By 1964, 1,230 degrees had been awarded American health education specialists,[16] and during the ten-year period from 1960 to 1970, 1,251 health education specialists were graduated from American and Canadian schools of public health. Making approximate correction for the overlap of years and non-American graduates, approximately 1,800 health educators are presumed to have graduated from accredited master's-level programs. For purposes of projection the current supply of professionally employed health education specialists is assumed to be 2,000.

Between 1960 and 1970, schools of public health graduated 1,144 health educators at the master's level and 107 at the doctoral level. In 1969–1970, 12 schools awarded 160 master's degrees, and as of January 1971 there were 106 other institutions offering programs of specialization in health education. Of these, 89 offered bachelor's degrees, 73 offered master's degrees, and 30 offered doctor's degrees. Correcting for the 33 foreign students awarded master's degrees by schools of public health in 1969–1970 and assuming approximately 10 graduates each for the six additional APHA-accredited schools that offer health education, approximately 190 master's graduates were produced that year from accredited programs. Projections for the remainder of the decade of the 1970s assume graduating classes of approximately 200 per year.

In 1966 a follow-up study was done of the 402 Americans who had earned a master's degree in health education at the University of North Carolina from the founding of the department through August 1966. Of the 320 on whom information could be obtained, nine were deceased, 46 were "retired" (usually women with young children), and 31 were in a field considered outside of but related to health education. The aforementioned 86 health educators represented 26.9 percent of the 320 for whom information was available. Since information was not available on 82 graduates, the true loss rate is probably significantly higher. Projected losses for the decade 1970–1980 assume a 1 percent annual attrition for new graduates and 1.5 percent for those employed in 1970.

Based on the above assumptions, the Task Force on Community Health Manpower projected the supply of professionally trained health education specialists in 1980 to be 3,610. If we extend these same assumptions for an additional five years, the projected number of health education specialists in 1985 would be approximately 4,350.

Requirements. The earliest projections for health education manpower were made in 1945 in the Haven Emerson Report,[17] in which one health education specialist (presumably with an MPH or MSPH degree) was recommended for each 50,000 population in local health department units. The criteria for the projection were related to the service setting and some sort of "service load" among nurses, sanitarians, and other professional personnel in the unit. If those criteria were applied today, there should be approximately 4,320 health educators in local health departments. The number currently so employed is unknown, but is generally believed to be no more than one quarter of that projected requirement.

Additional estimates have been made more recently, ranging from recommendations of one health education specialist per 9,000 population to one per 25,000, although again there is a lack of a clear rationale for these ratios. The Division of Manpower Intelligence of the Department of Health, Education, and Welfare has estimated a need for 4,000 professionally trained health educators by 1980 beyond those 2,000 estimated to be presently employed.[18]

According to Simonds, the manpower projection of a total of 6,000 public health education specialists required by 1980 was made likely in the absence of knowledge about major developments in the health sector that will make further demands on professionally prepared manpower, such as the following:

1. The movement in hospitals (7,000 member hospitals of the American Hospital Association) towards increased programming efforts in personal and community health education.
2. Initiation of reimbursement procedures so that health care facilities can be reimbursed by third-party payers for patient education services.
3. Inclusion of health education within the legislation for Health Maintenance Organizations.
4. Inclusion of health education as a basic function of regional health systems.
5. Potential inclusion of health education within national health insurance legislation.

It is likely, therefore, that the 6,000 figure is an underestimate. Although no adequate assessment of existing vacancies exists for health education manpower, it is evident from a recent study of job offerings that was reported in the *Journal of the American Public Health Association* that health education specialists at the MPH/MSPH level are among the most frequently sought-after professionals.[19]

Relating Supply to Requirements. Even if we assume an estimated requirement of 6,000 health education specialists in 1980 (and approximately 10,700 for 1985, if the same growth rate is extrapolated), the schools would have to increase their output from 200 per year to over 500 per year.

A forthcoming publication on health education manpower[20] indicates that serious gaps exist in present knowledge about health education manpower and that new studies must be undertaken. The number of health education tasks performed by other disciplines and the increasing use of health education manpower trained at baccalaureate levels for first-level positions are but two of the major developments in the field itself that affect total requirements. New groups of educators within the health care system, such as diabetes educators, indicate that the health and patient education function is spreading rapidly in the health care system.

24

New kinds of health education manpower are being considered for positions in hospitals and other health care facilities.

References

[1] John J. Hanlon, "An Ecologic View of Public Health," *American Journal of Public Health, 59*, No. 1 (January 1969).

[2] Scott K. Simonds, "Health Education Manpower," Appendix D, *Report of the Task Force on Consumer Health Education* (Task Force IV), The National Conference on Preventive Medicine, June 1975.

[3] J.M. Rosenstock and J.P. Kirscht, "Practice Implications," Health Education Monographs, *Journal of the Society for Public Health Education, 2*, no. 4 (Winter 1974).

[4] Lawrence Green, "Toward Cost/Benefit Evaluations of Health Education," paper presented to the President's Committee on Health Education, National Center for Health Education, 1974.

[5] J. Simmons (chairperson) and A.F. Skiff (reporter). "Report of the Committee on Manpower Education," *Proceedings: Federal Focus on Health Education*, Bureau of Health Education, Center for Disease Control, Atlanta, Ga., June 1974.

[6] *The Report of the President's Committee on Health Education*, Washington, D.C.: National Center for Health Education, 1972, p. 18.

[7] Simonds, *op. cit.*

[8] Rosemary M. Kent, "Professional Public Health Education National Manpower," testimony provided before the President's Committee on Health Education, Atlanta, Ga., January 27, 1972.

[9] U.S. Department of Health, Education, and Welfare, *Health Resources Statistics, 1972-1973*, Washington, D.C.: Government Printing Office, 1973, p. 159.

[10] Task Force on Professional Manpower for Community Health Programs (Thomas L. Hall, coordinator), *Professional Health Manpower for Community Health Programs*, Chapel Hill, N.C.: Department of Health Administration, School of Public Health, University of North Carolina, 1973, p. 52.

[11] *Ibid.*

[12] U.S. Department of Health, Education, and Welfare, *Health Resources Statistics, 1972-1973*, p. 159.

[13] *Ibid*, p. 159.

[14] *Ibid.*

[15] Simonds, *op. cit.*, p. 3.

[16] Kent, *op. cit.*, p. 1005.

[17] Haven Emerson, *Local Health Units for the Nation,* The Commonwealth Fund, 1945.

[18] U.S. Department of Health, Education, and Welfare, Public Health Service, NIH, Bureau of Health Manpower Education, Division of Manpower Intelligence, *Provisional Estimates*, Washington, D.C., 1972, p. 73.

[19] Task Force on Professional Health Manpower for Community Health Programs, *op. cit.*, p. 121.

[20] Scott K. Simonds, Robert Bowman, and Deanna Mechensky, "New Directions for Health Education Manpower Studies" (prepared for publication in 1975).

Tracer: Pharmacist

This tracer was prepared by Jere E. Goyan, PH.D.

Role. The pharmacist presently plays a very limited role as a provider of preventive services, although he has the potential for assuming a much more active part in this area. The easiest way to visualize this is to indicate on the provider/activity/target matrix both his current level of participation in certain key preventive health areas and his potential level.

Given the following areas of concern,
1. venereal disease,
2. family planning,
3. drug abuse,
4. cancer,
5. malnutrition, and
6. hypertension,

this is how the two matrices might look (placing a number from the list above in a cell of the matrix assumes that a significant number of practitioners presently take part in that activity); see Table 1.

Table 1.

| | PRESENT SITUATION | | |
| | Target | | |
ACTIVITY	Individual	Family	Community
Early diagnosis and treatment	3,5		
Health education and promotion	1,3	3	1,3
Health protection	1,3		3

| | POTENTIAL SITUATION | | |
| | Target | | |
ACTIVITY	Individual	Family	Community
Early diagnosis and treatment	1,3,4,5,6		
Health education and promotion	1,2,3,4,5,6	3	1,2,3,4,5,6
Health protection	1,3,5		3,4

Responsibilities and Functions. The pharmacist today rarely thinks of himself as being responsible for any preventive measures beyond, perhaps, making space available on a counter in his pharmacy for brochures on such subjects as diabetes, hypertension, and malnutrition. This is undoubtedly due to the low priority for—or, in most cases, total absence of—education in preventive medicine in schools of pharmacy. The past few years, however, have witnessed a surge of interest in several specific areas, among them venereal disease, hypertension, and diabetes. For example, in the last several years special issues of *Journal of the American Pharmceutical Association* have been devoted to the pharmacist's war on V.D., the identification and treatment of drug abuse, the challenge for pharmacists in helping to monitor and control high blood pressure, the pharmacist's involvement with special health problems (including family planning, suicide, and mental retardation), and patient record systems (as related to drug misuse).[1]

Groups of pharmacy students have instituted a number of programs in community health, including very active efforts in drug abuse education.[2] One California pharmacist was responsible for two V.D. "teach-ins" for high school and college instructors in northern California. The same pharmacist is currently supporting a hypertension clinic in his drugstore, using nursing and pharmacy students to screen customers. Many local pharmacy associations have instituted poison prevention campaigns, including distribution of syrup of ipecac and antidote charts to the public.[3]

A recent paper by M.C. Smith and J.T. Gibson speaks strongly to the potential roles of pharmacists in preventive medicine and identifies drug abuse, drug reactions and interactions, venereal disease, family planning, screening and diagnostic testing, immunizations, and nutrition as areas in which the pharmacist should be making contributions.[4] It is interesting to note, however, that a recent book on the social and behavioral aspects of pharmaceutical practice, that was coedited by one of the authors of the paper above, does not contain the term "preventive medicine" in its index.[5] This illustrates not only that little consideration has been given to the potential use of pharmacists in prevention by those within as well as those outside the profession, but also that even among those who have considered this potential, it seems to be regarded more as a theoretical goal than as an implementable objective.

*Factors Influencing the Participation of Pharmacists
in the Practice of Prevention*

1. Policy: Education for prevention in schools of pharmacy cannot be accomplished until there is recognition on the part of educators and/or legislators of the need for it.

27

2. Structure: The size, distribution, and relatively expensive education of the pharmaceutical corps (about 100,000 practitioners, who are geographically well dispersed and accessible) are among the strongest arguments for inclusion of the pharmacist in planning preventive strategies.

3. Interrelationships: The interrelationships of pharmacists with other members of the health care team have traditionally been tenuous. Recognition of the pharmacist as a potential provider by physicians, nurses, and others would be important to success.

4. Financing: If health education is not funded or reimbursed, it will not happen. Historically, pharmacists have rendered much "free service" (over-the-counter drug advice, home delivery of drugs, etc.); however, the continuing squeeze on the pharmacist's income is beginning to change even this situation, and it is highly unlikely that he would be willing to assume additional responsibilities in educational areas without pay.

Recommendations

1. In view of the fairly broad education of pharmacists—including biological, physical, clinical, and some behavioral sciences—it would seem that the primary deficiency in the education of the pharmacist for preventive medicine is the lack of an introductory course in the subject and some role models at the clinical level. To remedy this, not only should an introductory course in preventive medicine, including epidemiology, be offered (or perhaps even required) by schools of pharmacy, students should also have the opportunity to observe preventive medicine in action, preferably practiced by pharmacists. For example, Health Hazard Appraisal, as proposed by Dr. L. Robbins and co-workers,[6] could easily be performed in "corner drugstores."

2. A funding mechanism must be found if pharmacists are to be meaningfully involved in preventive medicine. Perhaps some form of capitation for pharmaceutical services that included preventive medicine efforts would be workable.

3. Pharmacists must be convinced that preventive medicine measures are meaningful in terms of patient outcomes. Like most other health professionals, the pharmacist is treatment-oriented and somewhat cynical about the potential benefits of preventive measures. Although it has many faults, a recent article by E. deHaas on system engineering and preventive medicine[7] is the type of argument that needs elaboration to health professionals.

Manpower Considerations. This section of the tracer was written by Thomas L. Hall, M.D..

As pointed out above, the pharmacy profession is often overlooked as an important resource for the early detection and referral of disease conditions, for patient education in the proper administration of drugs, and for the prevention of drug-caused disease. Various studies, such as that prepared by a recent Advisory Commission on Pharmacy in the State of California,[8] have recommended that pharmacists, in collaboration with other health care professionals, take a more active role in patient counseling and in the detection of potential problems of drug incompatibility and allergies. This section presents supply projections for pharmacists by way of indicating the large number of persons who will require strengthened training in the preventive and public health aspects of pharmacy.

Pharmacy training typically requires five years of study following graduation from high school and leads to a Bachelor of Science in Pharmacy or a Bachelor in Pharmacy degree. All schools now include some training in public health, though various authorities believe this aspect of pharmacy training should be further strengthened.[9] Most states require pharmacists applying for licensure to have completed an internship and to have performed satisfactorily on the state's examination, in addition to having had accredited professional training.

Present Supply. There were approximately 129,300 active pharmacists in the United States in 1970, of whom 9 percent were women.[10] The population per pharmacist varied from a low of 1,316 in the New England region to a high of 1,852 in the South Atlantic region, and by state from a low of 1,176 to a high of 3,703. The national average was 1,589, a slight deterioration from the average of 1,470 that prevailed in 1930. Over 80 percent of all pharmacists were working in community pharmacies, slightly less than 10 percent were in hospital pharmacies, and the balance distributed among manufacturing, teaching, government, and other activities. By 1973, the most recent year for which data are available, there were an estimated 132,899 active pharmacists.[11]

Projected Supply. The Bureau of Health Resources Development has prepared various projections of the supply of pharmacists at five-year intervals up to 1990. These presume no further additions to the number of pharmacy schools beyond the 73 in operation in 1972-1973, and make varying assumptions about the degree to which average school enrollments will continue to increase, about the percentage of women students, and about intraschool and postgraduate attrition. The "basic methodology" projection assumes that the annual number of graduates will increase about 50 percent during the 1970-1990 period (from close to 5,000 to almost 7,500). The total number of active pharmacists would thus climb to 179,900 for a 13 percent increase in the pharmacist: population ratio (1:1,393), though when converted to full-time equivalents this number would drop 5 percent to 171,000. The highest and lowest of the alternative estimates of the number of active pharmacists are 194,200 and 171,800, respectively. The basic projection anticipates a total input of new

29

graduates of almost 127,000 during the 20-year period, a number equal to the current supply of active pharmacists.

Requirements. No projections are available for the probable requirements of pharmacists. However, with no current evidence that pharmacists are having difficulty in finding employment, and with the projected annual increase in pharmacists exceeding the rate of population growth by only 0.71 percent, it is probably safe to presume that the projected supply will not exceed demand. Task Force V believes that if action were taken to decrease the high proportion of time (about 50 percent) that the average pharmacist spends on nonprofessional activities in the operation of a pharmacy, and if much of the time thereby saved were allocated to preventive and public health functions, the contribution the pharmaceutical profession could make to the health of the public would be very substantial.

References

[1] *Journal of the American Pharmaceutical Association, NS 13* (1973): 177; *ibid., NS 13* (1973): 665; *ibid., NS 14* (1974): 171; *ibid., NS 9* (1972): 453; *ibid., NS 13* (1973): 341.

[2] M. Martinetto, "Pharmacists in Community Health," *Journal of the American Pharmaceutical Association, NS 12* (1973): 700.

[3] M. Martinetto, "A Survey of Distribution Programs," *Journal of the American Pharmaceutical Association, NS 11* (1971): 8.

[4] M.C. Smith and J.T. Gibson, "The Pharmacist and Preventive Medicine," *Journal of the American Pharmaceutical Association, NS 15* (1975): 79.

[5] A.I. Wertheimer and M.C. Smith, *Pharmacy Practice: Social and Behavioral Aspects*, Baltimore, Md.: University Park Press, 1974.

[6] J.H. Hall, L.C. Robbins, and N.B. Gesner, "Whose Health Problem," *Postgraduate Medicine, 51* (1972): 114.

[7] E. deHaas, "System Engineering Applied to Health Care," *Transactions of the New York Academy of Sciences, 36* (1974): 613.

[8] *Report to the Speaker of the Assembly by the Advisory Commission on Pharmacy*, State of California, November 5, 1974.

[9] Melvin R. Gibson, "Public Health Education in Colleges of Pharmacy, III: The Testing Analysis of Tests, Conclusions, and Recommendations," *American Journal of Pharmaceutical Education, 37* (1973): 1.

[10] The primary source for this section is U.S. Department of Health, Education, and Welfare, Public Health Service, HRA, Bureau of Health Resources Development, *The Supply of Health Manpower: 1970 Profiles and Projections to 1990*, DHEW Publication No. (HRA) 75-38, December 1974, pp. 93–102.

[11] U.S. Department of Health, Education, and Welfare, *Health Resources Statistics: Health Manpower and Health Facilities, 1974*, DHEW Publication No. (HRA) 75-1509, Washing-

ton, D.C.: Public Health Service, 1974, pp. 243–253, provides information on the distribution of pharmacists and pharmacy students by state.

Tracer: Family Physician

This tracer was prepared by Thornton Bryan, M.D., and Michael M. Stewart, M.D.

Primary Care Physicians. The recent emergence of primary health care as a high national priority, together with the general assumption that primary care physicians will play a vital role in providing preventive services in the future, indicates the need for an analysis of the preventive tasks for which the primary care physician is to assume responsibility. At present, three major types of primary physicians are being trained: family physicians, general pediatricians, and general internists. These three types of "generalists" are technically specialists, in the sense that all are trained to board-eligibility level. What differentiates these primary care physicians from other clinical specialists and subspecialists is their major involvement in three functions: provision of accessible first-contact care, responsibility for longitudinal continuity in therapeutic management, and coordination integration of all health services required by the individual patient.

The Family Medicine Specialist. Family physicians currently constitute the largest identifiable group of primary care physicians. There are some 60,000 general practitioners and family physicians now active, including approximately 35,000 members of the American Academy of Family Physicians, of whom 7,000 have been certified by the American Board of Family Practice. In addition to performing the three characteristic functions of the primary care provider (first-contact care, therapeutic continuity, integration and coordination of services), family physicians are distinguished by their awareness of the effects of family make-up and of other psychosocial and environmental factors on health and disease. In the majority of cases, this family orientation also implies direct management or supervision of health and medical care problems for all members of the family group.

Family Physicians and Preventive Medicine. Family physicians are specifically concerned with health maintenance over time: their main focus is on the person rather than the disease, and on identification and modification of those factors that threaten the individual's health status. These efforts require longitudinal data collection in order to monitor health status, to identify the existence of risk factors, to detect disease at the preclinical stage, and to coordinate appropriate preventive and

31

therapeutic interventions. The training of family physicians should therefore include specific attention to:

1. *The health maintenance data base.* Initial acquisition and periodic updating of a data base for individual patients as an ongoing measurement of health status and as a means of risk-factor analysis.

2. *Validation of the data base.* Evaluation of the adequacy and utility of various methods of health-status and risk-factor analysis.

3. *Evaluation of outcomes.* Long-term assessment of the outcomes of various preventive interventions.

4. *Health team management.* Management of health care teams, with delegation of preventive tasks to physician extenders and other personnel, specifically including development of partnership relations with other primary care providers (nurse-practitioners, physicians' associates) in ongoing health maintenance as well as in therapeutic management of patients, particularly those with chronic disease.

Problems in Preventive Medicine Training of Family Physicians

1. Lack of a commonly accepted definition of primary health care, with identification and delineation of associated, effective health maintenance activities.

2. Failure to achieve proper integration of family medicine training activities with those of preventive/community medicine, due partly to the different perspectives and emphases created by separate educational programs in these disciplines. A simple schematic representation of the major focuses of these two areas of practice helps to visualize the problem.

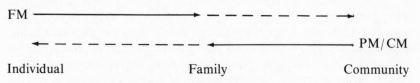

| Individual | Family | Community |

3. Predominantly didactic teaching of the basic skills of preventive medicine (such as epidemiology and biostatistics), with inadequate emphasis on the clinical application of these skills in family-oriented practice settings.

4. Inappropriate attitudes created in medical students by the common use of tertiary care as the major learning model. Development of the preventive attitude requires frequent and sustained exposure to the problems of health maintenance, early detection of disease, and preventive intervention.

5. A relative lack of emphasis on training the family physician for the role of primary health team leader, with responsibility for coordinat-

ing, delegating, and evaluating the performance and results of preventive medicine tasks.

Recommendations

1. Development of a commonly accepted definition of primary health care, specifying an appropriate range of preventive medicine objectives and activities, which are based on analysis of documented health care needs.

2. Development of curricular objectives and content that integrate the overlapping concerns of family practice and preventive medicine for the individual-family-community health care continuum.

3. Teaching the basic concepts and skills of preventive medicine to medical students in a less didactic and theoretical manner, with increased emphasis on the applications of these techniques in primary health care settings, serving a broad range of population groups.

4. Development of new training sites for family physicians, such as satellite health centers and Area Health Education Centers, where the dominant concern is primary health care delivery, specifically including the clinical practice of preventive medicine by health care teams.

5. Design and implementation of curricular objectives and content that enable family physicians to acquire the skills (interpersonal, administrative, planning, etc.) needed for effective health team leadership.

6. Emphasis on the collection of morbidity data from the ambulatory setting (as opposed to the mortality statistics so prevalent in epidemiology) to define more accurately the real preventive and therapeutic needs of primary care.

7. Preparing primary care physicians to work with community-based preventive health services, both in referring patients for care and in reporting information of epidemiologic significance. See Appendix B for a more detailed discussion of how this community-oriented role could be addressed in the education of primary care physicians. This goal would also be furthered by the accomplishment of Recommendation 4, above.

Manpower Considerations. This section of the tracer was written by Thomas L. Hall, M.D.

The educational requirements for family physicians include four years of medical school and three years in a family medicine residency. In 1972 there were 151 approved family medicine residency programs enrolling 1,041 physicians and graduating 919.[1] A survey conducted in 1973 by the American Academy of Family Physicians indicated that the number of approved programs had risen to 164, employing 1,754 residents.[2] That same survey revealed that 86 percent of first-year residency positions in family medicine had been filled—a healthy accomplishment for an emergent specialty.

The data on the total number of family physicians practicing in the United States are somewhat confusing because of the close association of family practice with the more traditional general practice. Although family practice has grown rapidly since its formal recognition in 1969, there has been a decline in the number of physicians who indicate that they function as general practitioners. This decline is reflected in the reported number of filled general practice residencies, which decreased from 925 in 1970 to 818 in 1972,[3] with a high proportion being filled by foreign medical graduates. Although some of the general practice training programs have been converted to family practice programs, others have been terminated.

Present Supply. At this time there is a discrepancy between the AMA statistics on family practice and those provided by the American Board for Family Practice (ABFP). According to the ABFP, 1,690 physicians became board-certified family practitioners in 1970, and 1,595 in 1971. The AMA figures for those years are 348 and 1,996, respectively.[4] The difference between the ABFP and AMA figures may reflect the mechanism used by the AMA in classifying practitioners according to the number of hours they report that they are working within a specialty. For example, an M.D. reporting 23 hours a week worked in internal medicine and 17 hours in family practice would be listed by the AMA as in internal medicine.

In any case, there were approximately 60,000 general and family practitioners in the United States in 1974. Of these, 35,000 were members of the Academy of Family Physicians, and approximately 7,000 had been certified by the ABFP.

Projected Supply. It is particularly difficult to develop projections of the future supply of family physicians, primarily because of the newness of the specialty and the uncertainty as to its future growth patterns. For example, using alternative planning assumptions to make projections of the future supply of physician manpower, the Department of Health, Education, and Welfare obtained greater variations in its projections of family physicians than in any of the other specialties. When the distribution of first-year residents in 1972 was used to determine the distribution of new entrants to the physician pool for the period 1970–1990, the projected supply of family physicians in 1980 and 1990 was only 6,610 and 12,630, respectively. These obvious underestimates result from the fact that 1972 was only the third year for family practice residencies and also from the fact that much of the present increase in family physicians is due to shifts out of general practice instead of only additions of new graduates. When alternative projections were made that did account for the growth in family practice residencies from 1970 to 1972 and did assume the continuation of that growth in the future, the projections for family physicians for 1980 and 1990 were 15,320 and 42,710, respectively. DHEW feels these latter projections should be viewed with considerable caution, due to the uncertainty of the future of family practice.[5]

The supply projections in Table 2 are made from several sources of data and should be used with discretion. The estimates for general practitioners are taken directly from estimates developed as part of "Project SOAR" (Supply, Output, and Requirements), and include a complex series of assumptions about additions and losses to that particular manpower pool.

The projections for family physicians are based primarily on data from the American Academy of Family Physicians (AAFP). They are offered as an alternative to the estimates derived by DHEW through Project SOAR that are reported above, which were based strictly on extrapolation of trends from 1970 to 1972. The AAFP has made projections of the growth in family practice residencies through 1985. They have made a high, low, and midline projection for each year; the midline has been used in Table 2. The AAFP also estimates that the percentage of residencies filled during that period will be approximately 90 to 95 percent, as it is at present. The additions for the projections below were developed using the AAFP estimates of graduates through 1977, and creating estimates from their projected filled residencies for the following year. The assumption of a 1 percent annual loss of both present family practitioners and new graduates is based on the newness of the specialty.

Requirements. It has been estimated by the American Academy of Family Physicians that the appropriate ratio of family physicians to

Table 2.   Supply Projections for Physicians in Family and General Practice in the United States for 1980 and 1985

YEAR		FAMILY	GENERAL	TOTAL
1975	Estimated number in practice	7,000	53,000	60,000
	Additions of family practitioners, 1975–1980	+ 8,455		
	1% annual loss of family practitioners, 1975–1980	− 502		
	Projected loss of general practitioners, 1975–1980		−17,010	
1980	Projected supply	14,953	45,990	60,943
	Additions of family practitioners, 1980–1985	+15,660		
	1% annual loss of family practitioners, 1980–1985	− 1,042		
	Projected loss of general practitioners, 1980–1985		− 5,000	
1985	Projected supply	29,571	40,990	70,561

population in the United States by 1985 should be 1:2,500.[6] If we assume a projected population of 230 million for the United States in 1985, the requirements for family physicians in that year would be 92,000.

Relation of Supply to Requirements. There is an apparent projected shortage of family and general practitioners in 1985 of approximately 22,000, if the projected supply of 70,561 is compared to the stated requirements of 92,000. This shortage is quite misleading, however, due to the role of pediatrics and internal medicine in the delivery of primary care. Depending on the assumptions, these two specialties alone will have a combined total of approximately 75,000 active physicians practicing in 1980, and this figure can be assumed to increase to approximately 90,000 by 1985. Thus, even if we assume that physicians in internal medicine and pediatrics cannot be substituted on a one-to-one basis for family physicians, the shortage implied by simply looking at family and general practitioners is not serious. Since the *supply* of primary care physicians is not the crucial issue in the more effective delivery of preventive care, then perhaps more attention should be given to the *training* of these physicians for prevention. The solution to the problem in the case of this manpower category seems to lie more in what kind of care is given than in finding more people to give it.

References

[1] AMA Council on Medical Education, *Directory of Internships and Residencies, 1973-1974,* p. 3.

[2] American Academy of Family Physicians, *Directory of Approved Family Practice Residencies, 1973-1974.*

[3] United States Department of Health, Education, and Welfare, Public Health Service, HRA, Bureau of Health Resources Development, *The Supply of Health Manpower: 1970 Profiles and Projections to 1990,* DHEW Publication No. (HRA) 75-38, Washington, D.C.: Government Printing Office, December 1974, p. 61.

[4] *Ibid.*

[5] *Ibid.* pp. 63-76.

[6] Personal communication with Dr. Robert Graham of the American Academy of Family Physicians.

An Assessment of Physicians' Attitudes Toward Prevention

This material on physicians' attitudes toward preventive endeavors has been prepared by John Colombotos, PH.D.

Any program that seeks to promote the practice of preventive medicine must take into account the knowledge, interests, and attitudes of potential practitioners toward that activity. The following discussion deals with medical practitioners, although many of the statements made here could also apply to other health care providers.

The practice of medicine in this country is oriented toward the diagnosis and treatment of disease, rather than toward its prevention. This orientation is reflected in how the overall health care system is organized and in its *incentives* (e.g., how practitioners are reimbursed for their services). On the level of the individual physician, it is reflected in the greater *professional satisfaction* and stimulation he or she derives from curative activities than from preventive endeavors and in his or her perception of the greater *medical value* of the former. (It is interesting to speculate on whether the imminent doctor surplus being forecasted by the Department of Health, Education, and Welfare will have any effect on the willingness of physicians to engage more fully in preventive practices. The guess of this Task Force is that even a widely acknowledged oversupply of physicians would have a negligible effect on their perception of being needed first and foremost for the more "vital" functions of diagnosis and treatment, unless there is a concurrent change in the priority prevention is given by medical school faculties, health care consumers, and third-party reimbursers.)

Studies of Physicians' Attitudes toward Preventive Medicine

Data documenting physicians' attitudes and practices in preventive medicine are available from two recent studies. One, by Coe and Brehm, provides fairly extensive information on the attitudes toward and practice of preventive medicine by a national sample of general practitioners and internists.[1]

A second study entitled "Physicians View Social Change in Medicine: Intragenerational and Intraprofessional Differences," currently being done at the Columbia University School of Public Health, is based on a national survey conducted in 1973 of the attitudes of medical students and physicians, including house staff, toward changes in the health care system and related issues.[2] Though attitudes toward preventive medicine were not a major focus of this study, information about this area was obtained from two questions in the questionnaire. Respondents were asked to "agree" or "disagree," and to indicate whether they did so "strongly" or simply "somewhat," with the following statements:

1. *Medical schools should put more emphasis on preventive medicine in their curricula.*

The responses to this question are only a rough indicator of attitudes toward the general concept of "preventive medicine," a concept that

37

means different things to different people. The survey did find, however, that respondents with a "broad" view of the physician's responsibility were more favorable toward preventive medicine than those with a "narrow" view. Specifically, those who agreed with the statement that "good medicine requires more than just treating people who come for care; it requires that doctors work in programs to improve social conditions" were more likely to be in favor of preventive medicine than those who disagreed with that statement.

2. *The medical value of annual health examinations for people who are not sick has been exaggerated.*

One must be cautious also about trying to infer too much about attitudes toward preventive medicine from the response to this question, since the value of annual examinations is a complex issue on which even people who are firmly committed to preventive medicine may disagree.

With these caveats in mind, we can examine the responses to these questions (see Table 3) and speculate about the implications for education and training for preventive medicine.

Both the Coe and Brehm study and the Columbia study show somewhat favorable physician attitudes toward the concept of "preventive medicine," especially as indicated by the fact that three-quarters of the physicians agree that more emphasis should be put on preventive medicine in medical schools.[3] (See Table 3.) One must keep in mind, however, that the distribution of responses to a survey question depends a great deal on its wording, and some proportion of this figure should probably be interpreted as "lip service."

The study by Coe and Brehm shows further that *younger* physicians (i.e., those who graduated from medical school since 1950) and *internists* have more favorable attitudes toward preventive medicine and are more likely to engage in preventive practices than older physicians (i.e., those who graduated before 1950) and general practitioners.[4]

In the Columbia study, however, internists and general practitioners are essentially similar in their attitudes toward the emphasis that should be placed on preventive medicine in medical schools (40 percent of each group agree strongly that more emphasis should be placed on preventive medicine in medical schools), but there is some variation among other specialties (60 percent of the psychiatrists agreed strongly with the statement, compared with 51 percent of the pediatricians, and 33 percent of the surgeons).

The setting in which practitioners work (i.e., whether they are hospital-based or are in solo practice, a partnership, a small group, or a large group), the amount of their income, and the percentage of their income paid in salary make no difference in their attitudes toward

38

Table 3. Physicians' and medical students' attitudes toward preventive medicine, by percentage distribution

STATEMENT AND RESPONSE (Total base)	MEDICAL STUDENTS Year in medical school				HOUSE STAFF[a] Year of training			SENIOR PHYSICIANS (5317) weighted (2713) unweighted
	1 (919)	2 (770)	3 (841)	4 (335)	1 (215)	2 (173)	3+ (501)	
1. Medical schools should put more emphasis on preventive medicine in their curricula.								
Agree strongly	46	38	31	37	38	39	28	40
Agree somewhat	45	50	47	47	47	48	53	33
Subtotal	91	88	88	84	85	87	81	73
Disagree somewhat	7	9	10	14	11	9	18	19
Disagree strongly	b	2	2	2	1	3	1	4
Subtotal	7	11	12	16	12	12	19	23
Don't know, no answer	1	1	1	1	2	0	1	4
Total	99	100	101	101	99	99	101	100
2. The medical value of annual medical examinations for people who are not sick has been exaggerated.								
Disagree strongly	42	38	32	25	21	15	9	16
Disagree somewhat	40	44	41	35	27	24	24	16
Subtotal	82	82	73	60	48	39	33	32
Agree somewhat	14	15	22	30	34	35	39	35
Agree strongly	2	2	4	9	17	26	26	35
Subtotal	16	17	26	39	51	61	65	68
Don't know, no answer	1	b	1	b	1	0	1	1
Total	99	99	100	99	100	100	99	101

[a]Includes only house staff who are graduates of U.S. medical schools.

[b]Indicates 0.5 percent or less.

Source: Reprinted with permission from Medical Care 13: 369–396, 1975

preventive medicine. Also, there is no variation in the Columbia study in physicians' responses about the value of an annual health examination according to their specialty, the setting in which they work, or the amount or form of their income.

More directly relevant to problems of education and training is information on the *development* of attitudes among medical students and house staff toward preventive medicine. We turn to these data next.

It is generally believed, and a few studies have shown, that during the course of their training, medical students become more "cynical," less "idealistic" (at least temporarily), and less "sensitive" to the social and psychological needs of their patients.[5] These changes possibly touch, but only indirectly, on students' attitudes toward preventive medicine.

If we compare medical students and house staff in the Columbia study according to the year of their training—and assuming that differences between these groups represent *changes* in individuals' attitudes over time rather than initial and persistent differences in the cohorts—we find a steady and sharp decline in favorable attitudes toward preventive medicine (see Table 3). The proportion of respondents who "strongly agree" that more emphasis should be put on preventive medicine in medical school curricula drops from 46 percent among first-year medical students to 28 percent among third-year residents; the proportion who believe that the value of annual health examinations has *not* been exaggerated drops even more sharply, from 82 percent among first-year medical students to 33 percent among third-year residents. (Consistent with these results, a doctoral research study being done by Audrey Gotsch in the Division of Sociomedical Sciences at the Columbia School of Public Health finds a similar pattern among dental students in their attitudes toward preventive dentistry.)

The overall results of evaluation studies of the effects on students' attitudes of programs in community medicine, primary care, ambulatory care, and comprehensive medicine—close kin to preventive medicine— offer little cause for optimism.[6] They show limited success, at best, in keeping students interested in primary care and community responsiveness, in the face of the more "glamorous" lures of highly specialized medicine, and purely curative endeavors. This was also substantiated by the Columbia study. The proportion of responding medical students who planned to see most of their patients on patient "self-referral" (roughly equivalent to "primary care") rather than on referral from other doctors dropped from 70 percent among first-year medical students to 38 percent among third-year residents.

Implications of These Findings for Educational Programs. Clearly, on the basis of the Columbia data, medical students and house staff finish their formal training with less positive attitudes toward preventive medicine than when they started. This information suggests that we should look at not only the *cognitive* objectives of teaching programs in preventive medicine, but also at their impact on relevant *attitudes* and values of their graduates.

Perhaps we ought to look at the *total* medical school environment—including clinical faculty, who stress diagnosis and treatment of unique and dramatic illnesses rather than prevention and health maintenance. One strategy for such an approach would be to include both faculty and students as the target, and to integrate preventive medicine with the teaching of traditional clinical medicine, rather than to administer small dosages of preventive medicine in an environment basically unsympathetic to its objectives.

This discussion thus far has concentrated on attitudes of *physicians-in-training* toward preventive medicine. Interest among physicians in actually *practicing* preventive medicine, however (that is, their *behavior*), may be influenced by factors other than their *attitudes* toward it. There are other aspects of the health care delivery system that may promote or inhibit preventive medicine—for instance, provisions and incentives for preventive medicine under national health insurance, the use of physicians' assistants and nurse-practitioners for doing more routine preventive measures, and practice arrangements (e.g., prepaid group practice). These factors might override the negative attitudes toward preventive medicine developed in professional training.

The failure of educational and training programs to respond to changes in the system was identified by the Task Force as the cause of a number of inadequacies in the training of many kinds of personnel for the practice of health care in general and preventive medicine in particular. The tracer analyses that precede, as well as those included in Appendix A, have highlighted some of the discrepancies thus created between what a student is taught and what he or she actually needs to know to function effectively in the practice setting.

Part IV will offer some suggestions for approaches to education and training that the Task Force believes would help ameliorate this situation.

References

[1] Rodney M. Coe and Henry P. Brehm, *Preventive Health Care for Adults,* New Haven, Conn.: College and University Press, 1972.

[2] For some early findings from this study, see John Colombotos, Corinne Kirchner, and Michael Millman, "Physicians View National Health Insurance: A National Study," *Medical Care, 13* (May 1975): 369–396.

[3] See Coe and Brehm, *op. cit.*, p. 77.

[4] Coe and Brehm, *op. cit.*, Chaps. 3 and 4.

[5] Leonard Eron, "The Effect of Medical Education on Attitudes: A Follow-up Study," in Helen Hofer Gee and Robert J. Glaser, eds., *The Ecology of the Medical Student,* Evanston, Illinois: Association of American Medical Colleges, October 15, 1957, p. 25.
Howard S. Becker and Blanche Geer, "The Fate of Idealism in Medical School," *American Sociological Review, 23* (February 1958): 50–56.

[6] Agnes G. Rezler, "Attitudes Change During Medical School: A Review of the Literature," *Journal of Medical Education, 49* (November 1974):1023–1030.
George G. Reader and Mary E.W. Goss, eds., *Comprehensive Medical Care and Teaching,* Ithaca, N.Y.: Cornell University Press, 1967.

Part III: Education and Training for the Specialty of Preventive Medicine

An Overview of The Needs for Physician Education in Preventive Medicine

This general statement of the need for increased financial support of physician training programs in prevention was written by William P. Richardson, M.D.

Although a number of categories of health professionals are involved in the implementation of preventive medicine practices either as their major professional responsibility or as a part of their participation in clinical care, progress in the development of new knowledge in prevention, the promotion of strong community programs of prevention, and the inclusion of a strong preventive orientation in primary clinical care will be determined in large measure by the participation and leadership of (1) physician specialists in preventive medicine, and (2) other prevention-minded physicians, particularly those who are considered primary care physicians. Since this is the case, it is essential that major attention be given to formats of educational programs appropriate for both preventive medicine specialists and primary care physicians and to the kinds of financial support necessary for their effective development and stable operation.

Educational Programs for Medical Specialists in Preventive Medicine

The American Board of Preventive Medicine certifies physicians in four categories: public health, aerospace medicine, occupational medicine, and general preventive medicine.

There has been a great deal of discussion in recent years about the generally unenthusiastic attitudes among medical students and within the medical profession towards preventive medicine as a career (see, for instance, the examination of students' and physicians' attitudes toward prevention in general in Part II of this report). It is true that there have been a number of unfilled positions for residents in approved programs in the specialty of preventive medicine. This has been particularly the case for public health and occupational medicine residencies.

Two circumstances, however, offer hope that this recruitment problem can be resolved. The first is the heightened social concern evident over the past several years among medical students. The most striking evidence

43

of this is the great increase in the number of graduates choosing family medicine and other forms of primary care as their field of practice. Coincident with this is a less pronounced but nevertheless heartening increase in the number who manifest an interest in preventive and community medicine.

This increase of interest in preventive medicine has been evident in what has happened with respect to residency programs in the specialty area of general preventive medicine. Although not all residencies in general preventive medicine have been filled, the fact is that during the period when a substantial number of general preventive residencies were receiving funds for support of residents, both the number of residents and the number of individuals applying for certification in the subspecialty increased substantially year by year. The fact that the number of residents is now declining coincides with the cut-off of financial support for trainees. The significance of this phenomenon appears to be that support for residents is crucial to adequate recruitment, and to the continued existence of a sufficient number of strong, educationally sound residency programs.

The question may be asked why this matter of financial support should be of greater importance to training programs for preventive medicine than it is in the case of clinical residencies, in answer to which three factors may be cited. First, preventive medicine has a requirement for an expensive academic year. Second, it is unusual for the experience component of the preventive medicine residency to involve the provision of services for which remuneration can be justified, as is generally the case in clinical residencies. Finally, if the preventive medicine resident has to borrow money to cover his educational years, repaying that debt out of his professional earnings may be a relatively greater financial strain on him than on the clinicians, since the majority of preventive medicine specialists occupy salaried positions, and the salary level is far below the average income of physicians in clinical practice.

It is self-evident that any program of support for residency programs must be broad enough to insure the education of an adequate number of physicians in each of the four subspecialty areas, and that it must have stability and continuity. Specific support is needed in the form of training grants for academic and residency programs in all four areas of preventive medicine, and there must be safeguards against the kind of sudden phase-out of support that has resulted in the recent inactivation of a number of general preventive medicine residency programs.

The vigorous development of general preventive medicine residency programs during the years of traineeship support is in contrast to the experiences of public health and occupational medicine residencies. Public health residencies, which have never received much traineeship support, have lagged, and occupational medicine residencies have dwindled almost to the vanishing point.

Programs in aerospace medicine present a somewhat different picture. Most of the physicians in this area have been trained in programs conducted by and for the armed forces, and these have generally prospered. The small number of residents recruited into the two university residency programs that currently exist has been totally inadequate to meet the needs of civilian air services, however. Traineeship support is needed to make possible the recruitment of the substantial number of physicians needed for this purpose.

Meeting the Needs of Primary Care Physicians in Preventive Medicine

Many observers of the preventive health care scene believe that the key to the effective incorporation of preventive philosophy and practice into the education and training of primary care physicians is strong, effective departments of preventive and community medicine. With the emphasis traditionally given to the clinical aspects of medicine and the generous support for research and training available to most clinical departments, departments of preventive medicine have only occasionally fared well enough in either status or support to mount the kinds of attractive, highly visible programs that have a significant impact on medical students.

A substantial level of additional support is essential. Federal grants to medical schools for education for prevention should, however, be provided only on the condition that a department or division should exist (or be created) which has interest in and specific curriculum responsibility for the preventive/community area and has sufficient autonomy to develop and carry out an effective program. Among the programs such support should make possible are:

1. Teaching of the sciences underlying preventive medicine and the preventive practices that should be a regular ingredient of clinical practice.

2. The inclusion of a strong, highly visible component of personal preventive measures in the medical care settings in which both medical students and house staff receive clinical experience.

3. The provision of elective clerkship opportunities in preventive medicine for medical students.

4. The development of continuing education in areas related to prevention for both practicing physicians and preventive medicine specialists.

45

Tracer: Occupational Medicine Specialist

This tracer was prepared by Irving R. Tabershaw, M.D.. Tracers for all categories of health personnel have not been prepared and this tracer is intended to be illustrative rather than representative of the preventive medicine subspecialties. Although the role of the aerospace medicine specialist is very similar to that of the occupational physician specialist, the preventive medicine specialists in public health and general preventive medicine do not adhere strictly to the patterns that will be described here.

This evaluation of the physician in occupational medicine as a prototype of the specialist certified by the American Board of Preventive Medicine is intended to trace both his role in the practice of preventive medicine and his relationships to the allied health professionals who are engaged in health maintenance. From this evaluation, deficiencies in the specialist's knowledge will be described, and the educational and training needs to remedy the deficiencies will be clarified.

Role. The provider/activity/target matrix is modified for this specialty by adding *industry* as a target population group. The individual and the workplace are the major foci of the occupational physician's activities. The occupational medicine specialist is, of course, only one of numerous health professionals who can and do provide preventive services to people in industrial settings. Other providers include other types of physicians, especially primary care physicians and trauma or orthopedic specialists; nurses, including practitioner's assistants, first-aiders, audiologists, and optometrists; industrial hygienists (e.g., safety engineers, toxicologists, transportation specialists, products liability experts, and regulatory affairs experts); health educators and health administrators; dentists; orthodontists; pharmacists; podiatrists; etc.

The occupational physician occasionally works alone in a particular industrial setting, in which case he either personally provides or makes outside referrals for many of the health care functions of the personnel listed above. Much more frequently, however, he works in conjunction with at least one, and more likely several, of these other health professionals and functions as coordinator of the services they provide. He also has the responsibility for actions regarding the health of individual workers within the industry that employs him, a responsibility that is increasingly being regulated by law (e.g., by the Occupational Safety and Health Act of 1970). The occupational specialist or other physician practicing in industry is more and more being held accountable (through lawsuits, for example), for invasion of privacy, lack of informed consent for exposure to hazards, negligence, etc.

Scope of Practice. Virtually all the health problems of ambulatory

46

working adults that can be managed by preventive methods can be addressed effectively within the framework of industry. The physician serving industry is adequately trained to carry out personally or supervise the following functions:

1. emergency treatment and continued follow-up for illness and injuries causally related to the work environment;

2. emergency care at work for illness and injuries not occupationally related;

3. control (with the assistance of industrial hygienists, safety engineers, etc.) of hazardous agents and environmental conditions at work;

4. the prevention of illness and accidents on the job;

5. physical examinations for employees upon entry to work and periodically thereafter (upon job transfer, return from illness or disability, etc., and for routine monitoring of employee health);

6. biological monitoring, particularly as specified by the Health and Safety Standards;

7. detection and treatment of health problems inimical to the employee's working capacity (alcohol or drug abuse, for example);

8. implementation of public health programs that can benefit the worker (e.g., hypertension and obesity control, immunizations);

9. health counseling, both individual and group, for personal health maintenance, use of protective equipment, instruction in safety measures, etc.; and

10. health administration (administrating workmen's compensation and group accident and health insurance plans, relationships with HMOs, etc.).

Discussion. The following points all indicate that there is an inadequately filled demand in the United States for preventive health services in the workplace.

1. Although there is a need for most of the program elements just described in nearly all industrial establishments, the most common and often the only service provided is emergency first aid for injured workers. The value of the other preventive services has been demonstrated, and great practical experience with many of these programs exists among occupational physicians and the allied health professionals working in industrial settings. This knowledge and experience is scattered, however, and has never been effectively correlated and communicated to all involved in maintaining and promoting worker health.

2. There are over 80 million workers in American industrial and business establishments. Many workers are concentrated in large companies, but the vast majority of the working population is distributed

among smaller organizations. The local physician who is contracted with to give on-call, fee-for-service care to workers in these smaller establishments frequently has no preparation for or interest in providing preventive occupational medical services.

3. The number of physicians in the specialty of occupational medicine is woefully inadequate. Although some 2,250 physicians in a recent AMA questionnaire indicated a primary interest in occupational preventive medicine, there were only 665 board-certified specialists in occupational medicine as of 1974.

4. The specialist is the basic resource of new knowledge and its application. Without his leadership, the practice of preventive medicine in industry degenerates into a hit-and-miss proposition and frequently is not carried out at all. This is indeed a sad state of affairs, particularly considering the ideal opportunity provided by the industrial setting for preventive services to reach a very large, readily identified, receptive, and almost captive population group.

5. The public has indicated through Congressional action that it is interested in worker health and that it is aware of the implications to community health of the manufacture, distribution, and transportation processes necessary to provide and disseminate the wide variety of goods which our society enjoys.

Recommendations for Education and Training

There is some need for the development of academic programs tailored to the educational needs of recent medical graduates wishing a career in occupational medicine. The greatest need, however, is for mechanisms that would permit both the continuing education of physicians already practicing in industry and the reeducation of mid-career professionals who wish to enter the field. Physicians in mid-career are often attracted to preventive medicine because of its intrinsic interest, its wide scope, its potential benefits for society, and its lifestyle. The mid-career physician has at present no practical way to broaden his educational base or to qualify as a specialist without great sacrifice. Modalities must be developed that would permit the physician to prepare for the specialty board examinations while continuing to practice. These might include short courses, syllabi for home study, self-assessment techniques, and field experience under qualified preceptors. These same methods would also permit the specialist to qualify for recertification and relicensure. (For a more detailed discussion of these suggestions, see the section below entitled "Recommendations for the Education and Training of the Preventive Medicine Specialist").

Manpower Considerations

Both papers in this section were written by Thomas L. Hall, M.D.

The following two papers deal with the quantitative needs for perhaps the three most critically required manpower categories for prevention—preventive medicine specialists, epidemiologists, and biostatisticians. With some exceptions, none of these three groups of health professionals has major responsibility for the actual *provision* of preventive health care; rather, they spend much of their time either teaching or determining that which will be taught to providers. In other words, they are chiefly responsible for the development and dissemination of the knowledge base for prevention.

Although the fields of biostatistics and epidemiology are not subspecialties in preventive medicine, they are so closely allied to that specialty that it seemed more appropriate to include a discussion of them in this part of the report than elsewhere.

Manpower Needs for the Medical Specialty of Preventive Medicine

Community, preventive, and social medicine have received increasing attention in recent years. The field was recognized as a medical specialty with the formation in 1949 of the American Board of Preventive Medicine and Public Health, a name shortened in 1952 to the American Board of Preventive Medicine. Initially certification was only in public health. The other three subspecialty areas were added later: aerospace medicine in 1953, occupational medicine in 1955, and general preventive medicine in 1961.

The 1974–1975 *Directory of Approved Residencies* lists the following number of residency programs in the several areas:

Aerospace medicine	4
Occupational medicine (academic)	4
Occupational medicine (in-plant)	19
Public health	23
General preventive medicine	25

The number of actual positions offered is not available for the past two years. Reports submitted January 1, 1972, to the AMA Council on Medical Education projected 423 residency positions for the 1973–1974 year and showed a total of 189 positions filled as of September 1, 1971. Reports submitted January 1, 1974, anticipated 220 residency positions to be filled in the 1974–1975 year, of which 137 were in general preventive medicine.

Several comments are in order. First, only about half of the reported number of offered positions have been filled. Positions offered tend to be geared to available support for residents and to the realities of recruiting; thus, training opportunities could readily be expanded if support and demand were increased.

Programs in the four areas differ in several respects. There are two civilian aerospace residencies, but to date the great majority of residents have been members of the armed forces and have been enrolled in one of the two training programs conducted by the armed forces. Support for aerospace residents has therefore posed little problem.

Only two of the currently approved academic programs in occupational medicine and six of the 19 in-plant programs are expected to have any residents in 1974–1975. Both the number of programs requesting approval and the number of residents have dropped drastically in the last two or three years, and it is clear that both support for residents and recruitment are acute problems in the area of occupational medicine.

Public health residencies cover only the two years of supervised experience, the required academic year being provided at an approved school of public health. Except for one program under the aegis of the Army, currently approved programs are located in state health departments. Both support for residents and recruitment present significant problems, but not so great as in occupational medicine.

General preventive medicine residencies are, with one or two exceptions, approved for three years, although the third year may be provided at another institution, usually a school of public health, rather than at the approved institution. Three of the currently approved programs are in agencies of the armed forces, one in a nonmilitary federal agency, twelve in departments of preventive and/or community medicine, and nine in schools of public health. Recruitment has not been a large problem and, during the period when traineeship grants were offered, support was not a major one either. With the discontinuance of traineeship grants, support is becoming a serious problem and will for many residencies be insuperable unless the grants are renewed or some other form of federal support provided.

Supply. In November 1967, the National Advisory Commission on Health Manpower was able to identify 4,933 physicians listing themselves as specialists in preventive medicine. Of this total number, most (1,714) listed their primary focus as occupational medicine, 1,619 identified themselves as engaged in public health, 941 were listed in general preventive medicine, and 659 listed their specialty as aerospace medicine.

Table 4 indicates the changes in numbers listing themselves as practitioners in the four subspecialty areas between 1967 and 1972. The significance of the decrease in general preventive medicine is not clear, but the fact that the group as a whole showed strong gains from 1967 to 1972, increasing by 2,240, is both significant and encouraging.

In 1967, out of a total of 302,500 active physicians in the United States, only 4,933 (1.6 percent) were in the four subspecialty areas of preventive medicine, of whom only 941 (0.3 percent) were in general preventive medicine. In 1972, of a total of approximately 321,000 active physicians, the percentage in preventive medicine as a whole had increased to 2.2 percent (7,173). Of those 7,173 physicians in the field, fewer than half are board-certified in the specialty. Table 6 below gives the numbers who had been certified in each subspecialty area by the American Board of Preventive Medicine as of December 1974. The figures, no doubt, include a substantial number who have died, retired, or are practicing in fields other than preventive medicine.

Requirements. It is exceedingly difficult to translate what are obviously significant needs into concrete figures, and there is often a great difference between need and effective demand. The comments and figures that follow are presented with full realization of their limitations.

Aerospace Medicine. A conference on training in aerospace medicine in 1968 undertook to project needs in the civilian area to 1975. It was agreed that military requirements would depend on the world military and political situation and that accurate estimates could not therefore be made. In the civilian area it was estimated that an annual input into the specialty of 18 to 20 physicians would be required. This is, of course, substantially in excess of the small number currently being trained in programs in civilian institutions.

Occupational Medicine. In an article in the April 1972 issue of *Occupational Health Nursing,* Edgar F. Seagle, Special Assistant to the Director of the National Institute for Occupational Safety and Health,

Table 4. Supply of Specialists in Preventive Medicine,
by Subspecialty, 1967 and 1972

	1967	1972	PERCENT CHANGE 1967–1972
Public Health	1,619	2,906	79.5
General Preventive Medicine	941	840	−10.8
Occupational Medicine	1,714	2,506	46.1
Aerospace Medicine	659	921	40
Total	4,933	7,173	45.5

Source: U.S. Department of Health, Education, and Welfare, *Health Resources Statistics, 1973–1974,* DHEW Publication No. (HRA) 75-1509. Washington, D.C.

projected a need for 3,000 occupational medicine physicians. Even if positions were created for just half this number, a great strengthening and expansion of educational programs would be necessary.

Public Health. Public health is the oldest subspecialty area of preventive medicine and has by far the largest number of certified specialists and probably the greatest number of practitioners. Estimates of the number of public health physicians are not available, but the number of physician positions in public health agencies that are vacant, filled on just an acting basis, or filled by nonphysicians is substantial. It is clear that the number of physicians presently completing public health residency training, 25 to 30 per year, will have to be significantly increased if the needs of the future are to be met.

General Preventive Medicine. This subspecialty includes physicians who serve in a variety of capacities. The largest numbers are epidemiologists and teachers in departments of preventive and community medicine and in schools of public health. A growing number are in demand in connection with the planning, development, evaluation, and administration of health care programs.

Studies of requirements and needs have been made for two categories, teachers of preventive medicine and epidemiologists. There is obviously some overlap. At a workshop of the Association of Teachers of Preventive Medicine in 1972, Dr. Kurt W. Deuschle estimated the requirements for manpower in the field of general preventive medicine.[1] The following three paragraphs are excerpted directly from his paper.

The U.S. Public Health Service recommends a minimum of six full-time faculty members for a department of preventive medicine of any medical school of 96 or more. The Saratoga Springs conference of the ATPM in 1963 recommended a minimum of two faculty members in each of 4-5 core areas in any "research department," (and we would anticipate that all academic departments would aim to be research departments). Thus, we might compromise at eight as a minimum faculty size and hope for ten as an average since the number of large departments will be included in the average which really function as schools of public health. The Project on Teaching of Preventive Medicine of the Institute for the Advancement of Medical Communication in 1963 found the average-size department of preventive medicine included 4.8 members, 52 percent having five or less. The National Advisory Commission on Health Manpower in 1967 found 136 physicians employed full time in medical schools, or about 1.4 for each school, meaning that about one preventive medicine faculty member out of four is a physician. If we assumed that the percentage of physicians in preventive medicine departments ought to increase to 40 percent as the emphasis changes from biostatistics to health care research, this would mean a need for about 2.5 preventive medicine physicians per department plus another 0.5 for those retiring in the next ten years, or about 300 for the nation. This would be 30 graduates per year for the next ten years or just about the rate at which we are presently producing them.

This figure is obviously much too incomplete and needs a number of revisions both upward and downward. Even though we like to think of a residency program as aimed primarily at producing new teachers and research people for departments of preventive and community medicine, in fact only a small percent of diplomates will probably end up in such departments. The same commission report in 1967 showed only 1 preventive medicine specialist in 7 was located in a medical school. Many more were working in health departments, the U.S. Public Health Service and schools of public health, industry and the armed forces. Assuming these areas will require replacement and hopefully a fair amount of expansion, it would seem that the number of trained general preventive medicine graduates needed in the next ten years would be 4–5 times the 300 estimated above on the basis of medical school needs alone.

On the other hand, the main source of preventive medicine specialists in the past has been from physicians who have trained as clinicians and then for one reason or another make a switch into the field of preventive medicine. For a long time to come this will continue to be a major route by which physicians enter our specialty, and probably this is a good thing. However, this again reduces our estimate of the number of trained preventive medicine physicians who can be absorbed out of residency programs, let us say by about 2/3, i.e., to about 450 in the next ten years or about 1-1/2 times as fast as they are now being turned out.

Projected Balance Between Supply and Requirements. In summary, the anticipated needs for specialists in all the areas of preventive medicine are substantially greater than will be met by the present output of academic and residency programs. It seems probable that output could be increased by 50 or even 100 percent without danger of producing a glut on the market.

Deuschle points to the fact that approximately 30 graduates per year are presently being produced in general preventive medicine. He cites this as being inadequate to meet the increasing demand for persons in this field. He further notes that a final factor that should be taken into account is the possibility that as board qualification becomes a more important criterion for employment, and as health care research becomes a more important component of service positions as well as academic ones, there will be a tendency for health department (public health) residencies to

53

merge with or cooperate with academic programs, making the medical school a more important source of trained public health personnel. This last possibility is very difficult to quantify even as a guess, but it is probably safe to assume that we could increase the number of trainees by between 50 and 100 percent without any danger of producing a glut of general preventive medicine specialists. All this, of course, is contingent upon the assumption that adequate financing will be available—which, as was indicated in the preceding papers, is much more problematic in preventive medicine than in clinical medicine, since the service produced is a "public good" rather than a private one (in the economic sense) and hence only can be paid for in the final analysis through tax levies. It is thus subject to the vagaries of the political process.

In the immediate future at least, it seems quite likely that the major problem will be to find recruits for residency programs rather than to find positions for graduates. This, in turn, will be contingent upon finding adequate financing for the program. Federal support for all preventive medicine-public health residencies in fiscal year 1971 totaled only $880,000, which was apportioned among 95 trainees, averaging $9,300 per trainee, including tuition and travel. This clearly comes nowhere near providing the number of traineeships needed to supply the national need; nor are the stipends high enough to compete with growing clinical residency salaries, subsidized as they are by third-party reimbursement schemes.

Manpower Needs for Epidemiologists and Biostatisticians

Few health specialties have as much potential to contribute to the health of the public in relation to the number of persons required as do epidemiology and biostatistics. As medical science has identified more and more environmental, nutritional, genetic, occupational, lifestyle, and other factors that influence health, it has become essential to use epidemiological and statistical techniques to identify their relative importance in determining health status and to assess the efficacy of alternative therapies. Only with such information can those actually responsible for the direct care of the population be reasonably effective. Unfortunately, the general recognition of this situation has not translated itself into corresponding actions to train the requisite number of specialists in these fields. In the early 1970s, it was estimated that the supply of each specialty was only slightly in excess of 1,000, or one specialist of each kind per 100 million dollars of health care expenditures, and of those in active practice, substantially less than half have doctoral-level specialty training and perhaps even fewer have a prior medical degree.[2]

By way of illustrating the price the nation must pay for giving so little attention to the scientific study of the distribution and determinants of disease, one author suggests that "at least a quarter of the $100 billion annual health care budget in the United States is wasteful, and without substantial changes both the absolute and proportional waste may be substantially higher in the future," [2] while another documents the very low percentage of epidemiology and disease control proposals (21 percent) and of health services research proposals (14 percent) that have been submitted recently (many by investigators with minimal disciplinary training).[3] In addition to these inefficiencies, the lack of adequate epidemiological and statistical training given in medical schools (and, for that matter, in other health professional schools) produces practitioners who are for the most part uncritical of conventional medical wisdom and limited in their abilities to judge what medicine can contribute to human welfare.[4]

Supply. The university of North Carolina manpower study, based on secondary sources, estimated the supply of employed epidemiologists with master's- or doctoral-level training at 1,000 in 1970 and at 1,100 for biostatisticians in 1971. The 1980 supply projections, based on observed and projected enrollments as of 1973, were 1,800 and 1,700, respectively.[6] Although these increases (7.2 percent annually for epidemiologists and 9.2 percent for biostatisticians) are well in excess of the annual population growth rate, the fact that the current supply is so far below the level of need and that most of those available at present are without full qualifications means that, at the present rate of training, the shortage will persist for many years. Other factors that tend to aggravate the supply picture are the relatively low salaries available in the health sector for specialists in these fields, which means that few physicians or others with advanced training in related fields are attracted to the training programs that do exist. The lack of master's-level graduates has, of course, limited the capacity of existing doctoral programs. (Fewer than 100 doctorates in these fields are awarded per year.) The average age of physician-epidemiologists is considerably above that of physicians in general, making their work life correspondingly shorter.

Requirements. The University of North Carolina Task Force projected the 1980 requirements for epidemiologists and biostatisticians at 2,000 and 2,500, respectively, which would result in shortfalls of 300 and 800.[7] These projections, especially that for epidemiologists, were based on very conservative standards and hence can be considered low. This is especially true if one takes into account that these projections include both master's- and doctoral-level specialists, whereas there is an increasing need for persons with a doctoral degree—now representing a small fraction of the total supply. By way of comparison, it is interesting to contrast the projected 1980 requirement of 2,000 epidemiologists that was established by the University of North Carolina group with the results of a far more detailed study by the recently reorganized Scottish National Health Service, which estimated a need for about 200 "community medical specialists," who are primarily medical epidemiologists, for a population of 5 million. Extrapolating this ratio to the United States would result in a requirement of 8,000 epidemiologists, four times the University of North Carolina estimate. White, using a somewhat different route of calculation from the UNC group, derives a "most conservative estimate" of 2,000 epidemiologists needed immediately.[9] He then goes on, as does Henderson in her paper, to develop various recommendations oriented towards increasing the supply of epidemiologists and biostatisticians in the near future. Although opinion may differ as to the precise magnitude of future requirements for these two specialties, this Task Force strongly endorses the view that the current supply is very inadequate in relation to the enormous potential that epidemiologists and biostatisticians have for increasing the effectiveness—through teaching, research, program planning, and program evaluation activities—of all health workers in the practice of preventive medicine.

References

[1] Kurt W. Deuschle, "Objectives of Graduate (Residency) Training in Community, Preventive and Social Medicine," ATPM Workshop Conference, February, 1972, p. 11.

[2] Task Force on Professional Health Manpower for Community Health Programs (Thomas L. Hall, coordinator), *Professional Health Manpower for Community Health Programs, 1973*, Chapel Hill, N.C.: University of North Carolina, School of Public Health, Department of Health Administration, 1973, pp. 49, 67.

[3] Kerr L. White, "Opportunities and Needs for Epidemiology and Health Statistics in the United States," a paper presented at the Conference on Epidemiology as the fundamental basis for planning, administration, and evaluation of health services, Baltimore, Md., March 2-4, 1975, p. 8, which gives references to the estimate made by Sidney Wolfe at the DHEW Conference on Inflation (September 19-20, 1974).

[4] Maureen Henderson, "Needs and Resources for Epidemiology and Health Statistics in the United States," a paper presented at the Conference on Epidemiology *op. cit.*, pp. 12-13.

[5] Based on White, *op. cit.*, p. 6. Moreover, according to a survey conducted by W. H. Barker and reported in the *Association of Teachers of Preventive Medicine Newsletter, 21*, no. 1 (Spring 1974), only 75 percent of the medical schools in the United States in 1974 required at least one course in epidemiology. Furthermore, most such required courses simply provide descriptive material, giving students little insight into the problem-solving capacities of the discipline.

[6] Task Force on Professional Health Manpower for Community Health Programs, *op. cit.*

[7] *Ibid.*

[8] Scottish Home and Health Department, *Community Medicine in Scotland,* Edinburgh: Her Majesty's Stationery Office, 1973 (as cited in White, *op. cit.,* p. 14).

[9] White, *op. cit.*

Recommendations for the Education and Training of the Preventive Medicine Specialist

This section of the report was written by Raymond Seltser, M.D., M.P.H.

The process of *educating* professionals for work in the field of preventive medicine involves the acquisition of a body of knowledge and a familiarity with methods and procedures that are oriented more toward populations than toward individuals. Many preventive measures are related to the mass phenomenon of disease in some way—particularly as regards the type of measures applied in the "practice of preventive medicine" in the "field." Examples of this range from immunization procedures and the behavioral modifications involved in altering dietary patterns and smoking habits—as applied to individuals and groups of individuals—to restrictions of noise levels, purification of air and water, and institution of plant safety programs—as applied to the environment in which these groups of individuals operate.

The process of *training* individuals for work in the field of preventive medicine involves the acquisition of specific skills needed to prevent disease. Examples are the techniques of immunization, the conducting of field surveys to detect levels of air pollutants in various parts of a region, the conducting of smoking cessation clinics, and the carrying out of plant safety inspections.

The difference between "education" and "training" is more than a semantic one in the context of the deliberations of this Task Force. The settings in which these two activities are best conducted are different, and it is the recognition of this fact that suggests the need for adopting a strategy for educating that is different from that for training.

Education for Preventive Medicine

The objectives of an educational program for the field of preventive medicine should be based on a model which incorporates the following elements:

1. academic experience in an environment that has the potential for imparting a body of knowledge encompassing, at a minimum, the areas of statistics and epidemiology, environmental health science, health services administration, and behavioral sciences;

57

2. mechanisms for continually bringing preventive medicine practitioners up-to-date as regards both the expanding body of knowledge and the new methods and procedures that are being developed with the passage of time;

3. incentives to ensure the participation of practitioners in continuing education programs;

4. mechanisms for the initial education of mid-career professionals, providing basic knowledge of the essentials of environmental health science, biometry and epidemiology, and health services administration in nontraditional academic settings (i.e., on-the-job *education* as opposed to on-the-job *training*);

5. input into the academic environment of the continually changing problems of the "outside world" in which preventive medicine practices are applied.

Preventive medicine has been recognized as a medical specialty since the establishment of the American Board of Preventive Medicine in 1948. Originally established to certify specialists in the field of public health, there has been a gradual evolution resulting in the Board's now certifying specialists in four areas of preventive medicine: public health, aerospace medicine, occupational medicine, and general preventive medicine. As of December 1974, a total of 3,390 individuals had been certified as specialists by the Board. Tables 5 and 6 help to visualize the numerical relationships between physicians in other specialties that have a major involvement in the provision of preventive medical care and those in the actual specialty of preventive medicine (Table 5), and among physicians certified in the four areas of that specialty (Table 6).

The policy of the Board has been to develop guidelines for education and training within the four areas of preventive medicine. It is useful to

Table 5. Manpower in Preventive Medicine and Primary Care Specialties, December 1972

SPECIALTY	ALL PHYSICIANS NOT IN TRAINING	NUMBER CERTIFIED	PERCENTAGE CERTIFIED
Preventive Medicine	7,025[a]	2,262	32
Family/general practice	54,322	4,542	8
Internal medicine	46,610	22,851	49
Pediatrics	16,277	13,214	81
Obstetrics-gynecology	17,146	11,409	67
Total primary care physicians	134,355	52,016	39
All physicians	302,983	136,406	45

[a]This figure does not correspond with the figure of 7,173 given for the same year in Table 2, as that figure *does* include physicians in training.

Source: Annual Report of the American Board of Medical Specialties, 1972-1973.

Table 6. Board-Certified Physicians in Preventive Medicine, by Area of Specialty, December 1974

AREA OF SPECIALTY	NUMBER CERTIFIED
Public health	1,752
Aerospace medicine	693
Occupational medicine	665
General preventive medicine[a]	280
Total	3,390

[a]It should be pointed out that the small number certified in general preventive medicine is somewhat misleading because many of those certified initially in public health were actually practicing in areas now identified as general preventive medicine, epidemiology, etc.

Source: U.S. Department of Health, Education, and Welfare, *Health Resources Statistics, 1973–1974*, DHEW Publication No. (HRA) 75-1509, Washington, D.C.: Government Printing Office, 1974.

compare the educational component of the requirements mandated by the Board to the five points in the model previously described. All of the following assume an accredited M.D. degree as a starting point.

1. There is an academic year built into the eligibility requirements of each of the four areas of specialization. However, in two areas—occupational medicine and aerospace medicine—experience in the field may be substituted for academic experience, although using this route takes considerably longer to satisfy minimum board-eligibility requirements. The essential elements of the academic program specify biostatistics and epidemiology, health administration, and environmental health.

2. The American Board of Preventive Medicine has committed itself to the development of a recertification program, in line with a similar commitment by all 22 specialty boards represented on the American Board of Medical Specialties (see Appendix C for their "Recommended Guidelines on Recertification for Specialty Boards"). This program is in the process of evolution, and specific recommendations for the form it should take will be introduced later in this paper.

3. Up to now there have been no incentives to ensure the participation of preventive medicine specialists in continuing education programs. In fact, the stimulus for a sudden intense interest in the development of such continuation education has come largely from practitioners in those states where *relicensure* of physicians is being tied to a requirement for the accumulation of a certain number of continuation education credits in the form of involvement with some organized academic-type experience. It is important to note that this affects all practitioners, not only certified specialists. This has led to the realization that it would make sense for the continuing education activities that are developed in response to the need for *recertification* of specialists to be identical to or, at least, coordinated with those developed in response to the needs for relicensure.

The ultimate objectives of the American Board of Preventive Medicine is to upgrade and maintain at as high a level as possible the competency of the practitioners of preventive medicine. (Board certification was never intended to be a *requirement* for the practice of a specialty, but rather a visible *recognition* by a group of peers of the attainment of a certain high level of proficiency in the practice of that particular specialty.) The Board recognizes its responsibility for developing both eligibility criteria and certifying examinations to enable practitioners who choose to do so to reach the objective of board certification. It also recognizes, however, that the development of continuing education programs geared only to certified specialists would be a great disservice to the majority of colleagues who are practicing preventive medicine without certification. (Board certification presently is held by only 32 percent of the total number of physicians listed in the AMA Directory as specializing in preventive medicine.) Therefore, the Board has requested that the professional societies, whose membership encompasses both board-certified and not board-certified practitioners, assume responsibility for the development of suitable programs of continuing education to meet the needs of their constituents. Since the American College of Preventive Medicine is the one professional society whose membership encompasses all four specialty areas, it is the logical organization to assume the leadership and coordinating role in implementing this proposed program.

The incentives for participation in a continuing education program can be categorized in the following manner:

a. Incentives already present and impelling: The relicensure requirement, already in force in several of the states, that is destined to become a more general requirement throughout the country.

b. Incentives soon to become a reality: Recertification by the American Board of Preventive Medicine is almost certain to be tied to a continuing education program developed by the professional societies.

c. Incentives which should be considered for implementation by the professional societies: Fellowship in the American College of Preventive Medicine is open to board-certified specialists of several boards other than that of preventive medicine (viz., internal medicine, pediatrics, and family practice), who are devoting themselves to the practice of preventive medicine. Continuation of fellowship status in the College could be made contingent upon participation in self-assessment examinations developed by the College. If these self-assessment exams were developed in conjunction with a series of syllabi that contained the answers to the exam questions, and if the only requirement were completion of the exam, with no necessity for attaining any stated grade level, we would have achieved the underlying purpose of initiating a continuing education program to expose and reexpose practitioners to new and fundamental concepts in their field.

The Board should also give consideration to coordinating the content of the self-assessment examinations with the certifying examinations. I would propose that the subject matter that is covered in the syllabi developed by the professional societies and used for the formulation of specific questions in the self-assessment exam in any given year comprise the subject material for, say, 75 percent of all questions contained in Part II of the board certifying examinations of the subsequent year. This might encourage a number of potentially board-qualified individuals to "risk" taking the formal examinations required for board certification.

Also, as previously mentioned, the Board should build its recertification program around participation in these proposed ongoing self-assessment continuing education programs of the specialty societies. Recertification should be voluntary for all present diplomates, but all diplomates should be required to participate in the self-assessment program of the College (or of their respective specialty society) at least once every four years, and to repeat Part II of his or her specialty area certifying exam at least once every six years. Failure to obtain a passing score on the Part II exam would mean an obligation to participate in the self-assessment exam program annually until successfully passing Part II any time within the following six years. The worst penalty that could be imposed, therefore, would be the requirement to participate in a continuing education program each year.

4. Schools of public health have been the traditional milieu in which mid-career professionals have obtained their initial educational experience in preventive medicine. The necessary exposure to biometry and epidemiology, environmental health science, behavioral sciences, and health services administration can be obtained in these schools, generally requiring a nine-month period of residence away from a job. There are many benefits to be derived from an educational experience in an academic setting on a full-time basis. However, both the times and the economy have so changed that the probability that large numbers of physicians will ever again be willing or able to take the necessary time off to receive full-time education and training becomes more remote with each presidential budget submission. On the other hand, the need for mid-career academic exposure is growing, requiring that new kinds of educational programs be developed if physicians are to continue to play a leading role in the practice of the preventive medicine and public health of the future. New patterns of funding must also be provided—and the logical route would appear to be something that is *not* dependent on federal funding. I suggest that one alternative is the development of an on-the-job educational program, in which opportunities are provided for physicians to take either refresher courses or introductory courses in the core areas of biometry, epidemiology, environmental health, and health administration, and possibly in the behavioral sciences. Innovative,

experimental programs initiated by schools of public health in recent years have attempted to provide such an "out-reach" service, especially for health department personnel. Funding problems have plagued these efforts, however, and the government has not been overly supportive (although certain *individuals* in government have been enthusiastic and therefore as frustrated by the lack of governmental support as their academic counterparts). It is suggested that there is a great need in industry at this time for this type of training—and the time may be right for the initiation of an effort in this area. (See Tracer: Occupational Medicine Specialist, Part II, for a substantiation of this suggestion.)

5. The extent to which the sites used for postgraduate education of preventive medicine specialists adequately reflect the actual practice conditions and problems of the "outside world" where preventive medicine practices are applied has recently been the subject of some exploration, particularly regarding the traditional use of schools of public health as the major educational site for such training. This is currently under study by the Milbank Foundation's Commission for the Study of Graduate Education in Public Health, and it is likely that some relevant comments on this point may be forthcoming prior to the time of the National Conference on Preventive Medicine in June. In addition to any recommendations that this commission may make, however, the previously mentioned plan of having syllabi and self-assessment examinations prepared under the direction of the professional societies would provide at least some feedback, which would ensure more adequate input from the outside world than in existing graduate programs.

Training of Physicians in Preventive Medicine

For the purposes of this paper, "training" can be defined as the development of expertise in applying the various techniques associated with the practice of preventive medicine. In the case of the physician preventive medicine specialist, the training period can be equated with that portion of a formal residency program which usually follows the academic period. This training generally consists of one or two years of supervised work in a wide variety of settings, ranging from the academic environments of schools of public health and medical schools to such operating units as health departments, industrial plants, and federal agencies.

The critical question that should be asked in reference to training is: What should specialists in the various specialty areas of preventive medicine be able to *do* once they have completed their training period? Logic dictates that this question should be answered before determining both the content of the training program and the minimum duration of the training period. It is disturbing to find how diverse are the points of view on this question within the specialty of preventive medicine, but the problem seems to be concentrated in the specialty area of general preventive medicine. (This newest of the specialty areas has been the most rapidly growing and is certainly the most difficult to define in terms of "what do specialists do?" It is also the least well understood area within the specialty itself.)

It would be inappropriate to attempt to detail in this paper the specifics of a training program for each of the areas of preventive medicine. However, the following five-step general approach can be proposed for the delineation and evaluation of training programs for preventive medicine, which would apply to all four of the specialty areas:

1. Define the range of specific competencies that is expected of individuals completing a training program in the particular specialty area of preventive medicine.
2. Define the nature of the training program that would provide opportunities to develop those competencies.
3. Define the minimum time period needed to provide opportunities for the development of these competencies.
4. Review existing (residency) training programs to determine the degree to which they *do* provide opportunities for the development of these competencies.
5. Develop methods of evaluating (by residency program directors) the extent to which their residents *have* developed in these areas.

In order to move in this direction, one of the existing bodies charged with responsibility for training in preventive medicine must assume some leadership in initiating the development of the first three steps in the above-described model. The American Board of Preventive Medicine and/or the Residency Review Committee for Preventive Medicine would seem to be the logical nominees for such a role.

The initial step could be the development of an evaluation document aimed at laying the foundation for assessing the competency of preventive medicine practitioners, which could be drawn along the lines of a similar document recently developed for the profession of pediatrics under the leadership of the American Board of Pediatrics. The general purpose of developing such an evaluation document would be to present in an organized manner a list of performance capabilities that could function as a blueprint for evaluating physicians who seek certification by the American Board of Preventive Medicine. Such a document should also serve the following more specific purposes:

1. It should provide the basis for the development of evaluation instruments which will (a) accurately measure the competence of

preventive medicine practitioners, and (b) point the way to developing new methods of evaluation.

2. It should serve as a guide to residency program directors in designing educational programs.

3. It should serve as a guide to residency review committees or other groups in developing standards for approval of training programs.

4. It should provide a guide to students preparing for careers in medicine.

5. It should provide a guide for the development of continuing education programs.

6. It should serve as a guide to practicing preventive medicine specialists as to how they can engage in a process of self-evaluation to maintain their knowledge and skills at adequate levels.

7. It should aid in identifying aspects of preventive medicine that can be assigned to individuals whose training differs from that of the preventive medicine specialist, such as primary care physicians, public health nurses, dentists, and health educators.

Part IV: Recommendations and Strategies for Change

Major Findings

All categories of health manpower, as well as policy makers and the public, are involved in prevention in its broadest sense. Task Force V approached the question of education and training for prevention through consideration of four major issues:

1. The range and types of activities that constitute preventive health care;
2. The various settings in which these preventive activities take place;
3. The different categories of health workers that are directly involved in providing preventive activities;
4. The types of education and training programs that are required to prepare various categories of health workers in sufficient numbers for effective provision of preventive health services.

Although it was unanimously agreed that prevention is not the exclusive responsibility of specialists in preventive medicine, nevertheless there are certain aspects of prevention that require the leadership and expertise of physicians and other health professionals who concentrate on prevention as their chief professional interest.

A careful analysis of the roles and functions of various categories of health workers in providing preventive services raises important questions about the adequacy of existing training programs:

1. Are the objectives of existing training programs consistent with the preventive roles for which health workers are being prepared?
2. Does the existing knowledge base provide sufficient educational content for training programs in prevention? Is this knowledge base effectively utilized?
3. Are the institutions responsible for education and training in prevention organized so as to make best use of available educational resources and learning sites?
4. How do institutional and governmental policy, structure, financing mechanisms and interrelationships affect current efforts in education and training for prevention?
5. Are existing programs in education and training for prevention adequate for meeting current and future manpower needs?

Task Force V has identified five general areas related to education and training for prevention in which changes are required.

I. The modification and strengthening of education and training programs so as to provide the specific competencies needed by health personnel to function effectively in different health care settings;

II. The way in which learning settings are managed, i.e., the structure and use of the academic and training environment;

III. The development and dissemination of the knowledge base necessary to support effective education for prevention.

IV. The development of educational and training continuums corresponding to planned steps in professional development.

V. The relationship of manpower needs for prevention to education and training requirements.

Permeating each of these problem areas is the magnitude and urgency of the need for support of educational programs to develop the essential manpower required. The short-term need is acute; current programs must be supported and expanded to insure continued availability of leaders in the field, i.e., as teachers, researchers, and practitioners. Addressing the long-term need also depends on meeting this immediate requirement, so that personnel will be available to staff programs now being enacted into federal legislation, such as OSHA and the National Health Planning and Resources Development Act of 1974 (P.L. 93-641). In particular, the impact of the failure of third-party payers to reimburse patient care programs for preventive services and the funding requirements for developing and maintaining high quality training programs must be recognized. Federal and private sector funding mechanisms must be established to provide for these preventive health manpower educational activities.

The Modification and Strengthening of Education and Training Programs so as to Provide the Specific Competencies Needed by Health Personnel to Function Effectively in Different Health Care Settings

Proposition. There are widespread deficiencies in educational and training programs for prevention, so much so that these programs present a weak base for launching a national program of prevention. These deficiencies stem from several sources:

1. inadequate importance given to prevention in federal legislation dealing with health care and manpower;

2. lack of priority given to prevention in educational and training programs for health personnel;

3. inadequacies in educational content and teaching methods relating to prevention, particularly the lack of close relevance between

66

educational programs and the competencies needed to be effective in current and projected preventive roles in health care;

4. inadequacies in the organization and management of settings for learning prevention (see Section II, below, on the management of learning settings);

5. insufficient funds to support education and educational research for prevention.

Major changes are required on the part of the federal government, educational institutions, and the health professions if there are to be meaningful changes in education and training for prevention.

Substantiation. Federal legislation related to health has a powerful impact on education and practice. Although prevention has been given prominence in some legislation, such as that relating to health maintenance organizations, early periodic screening of children, and the recently enacted National Health Planning and Resources Development Act, which identified prevention as one of the top priorities in health, other crucial proposals for health legislation almost completely ignore prevention. A number of current health manpower proposals, for instance, make almost no note of the need for preventive content in education and training programs, except through the important provisions for support of specific manpower categories and certain types of institutions, such as schools of public health (though even that support has been recommended for termination by the Administration). There should be much broader support for education for prevention, including requirements for preventive content in the curricula for all health personnel, that would match the explicit commitments to prevention that are now beginning to appear in some health legislation.

The preventive *content* of educational and training programs for all the health professions needs careful and systematic review. In some instances it is almost completely lacking, as in pharmacy; in others it is submerged by the predominance of other emphases, as in the relentless attention given to acute clinical problems in most medical curricula.

The greatest need is for careful analysis of the possible points of preventive intervention by various health personnel in various practice settings, and for the incorporation into educational programs of those learning experiences that will make personnel more effective in developing and implementing preventive policies in those work settings. (Indeed, the function of the "tracer" method used by the Task Force was to illuminate the discrepancies between educational preparation and practice needs.) Such an analysis could lead to the development of competency-based educational objectives that could be used both for the design and implementation of educational experiences closely related to operational settings and for the subsequent evaluation of such programs.

One suggested approach to analyzing and evaluating educational and training programs for prevention is outlined earlier in this report. Another approach is that taken by the Center for Educational Development in Health at Harvard University in Collaboration with the Association of Teachers of Preventive Medicine, a project to develop a competency-based curriculum for teaching preventive medicine to medical students (see Appendix C).

Beyond the specific content deficiencies revealed by the Task Force's analyses, a number of process skills that need to be kept in mind in developing and/or evaluating education and training programs for prevention were identified:

1. A need for problem-oriented rather than topic- or discipline-oriented teaching. In addition, the problems should be largely based on or taken from actual practice settings in the health care system.

2. A need for the development of skills both in team leadership and management, and in collaborating with other members of the health care team and with community groups and political forces.

3. A need for better role models. Because students' attitudes are influenced at least as much by the actions of their preceptors and instructors and by the learning environment as by curriculum content, it is important that teachers of health personnel be themselves committed to and actively involved in preventive activities.

4. A need for the development of skills in program evaluation and self-assessment.

Recommendations

1. That professional societies and educational institutions undertake a systematic analysis of the potential points of preventive intervention by various health personnel in different health care settings, and accordingly develop learning experiences that will make the professionals thus trained more effective in planning, implementing, and evaluating preventive activities and programs in those settings.

2. That the Fogarty International Center provide leadership in such efforts by convening an ongoing working group, including interested organizations, institutions, and individuals, to undertake a systematic examination of existing and potential applications of preventive measures in various medical and health care settings. That the results of this analysis be used as the basis for proposed changes in the education and training of various categories of health personnel, leading toward more widespread use of competency-based educational objectives and programs.

3. That federal legislation relating to health care and health manpower include more specific attention to prevention, including strong

encouragement of a preventive emphasis in the basic curricula for all health personnel.

4. That specific provision be made in federal health manpower legislation to provide career-development support for training of educational planners, developers, and teachers of prevention and prevention-related subjects for various categories of health personnel.

5. That federal and other support for primary care training programs for medical and nursing students, house staff, and physician extenders (including nurse-practitioners) require or encourage that educational objectives and processes relating to prevention be specifically included in those programs.

Management of the Learning Setting

Proposition. The way in which education and training programs for prevention are structured in educational institutions and the relationships they have with operational programs in the health care system are of great importance. The importance of internal institutional arrangements lies chiefly in the need for institution-wide, interdisciplinary planning and programming that would permit an efficient, integrated incorporation of preventive content into all health sciences curricula. External relationships with the health care system are important because so much of the effectiveness of health personnel in preventive programs depends on the structure, policies, and programs of the health care institutions and agencies within which they work and on their capability for adapting to or changing those situations. The challenge is to conceptualize, structure, and manage learning settings that prepare students to function effectively in real-world operational settings.

Substantiation. In many health sciences educational centers, preventive content is minimal or missing from curricula of a number of health professional programs. In addition, the resources for education in prevention that do exist, as in departments of preventive medicine and schools of public health, are often not widely appreciated or used. At times there is even duplication of these scarce resources. There is a clear need, therefore, for planning educational and training programs for prevention so as to take into account the needs of *all* health professional programs and to make best use of limited educational resources. This suggests the wisdom of designating *a preventive education resource group* in each health sciences center, which could include epidemiologists, biostatisticians, health educators, specialists in preventive medicine, health care administrators, etc., who could work in close conjunction with departments or schools primarily responsible for specific professional educational programs, assisting in the development of core courses,

69

teaching basic courses, and providing advanced learning experiences. The effectiveness of the preventive effort will depend largely on how these relationships within the institution are structured and managed and on the priority given to prevention by the institutional leadership and faculty.

External relationships with the health care setting are fully as crucial as the internal programs and priorities of the educational institution. The health care system has structural, functional, and policy components that often discourage or are actual obstacles to preventive activities. Personnel who have been trained exclusively in the theoretical aspects of prevention may be rendered ineffective in the work setting. It is necessary, therefore, that educational and training programs have close working relationships with operational health care programs in which students can learn how to cope with obstacles to their major functions and in which instructors and administrators of educational and training programs can themselves learn how such problems can be dealt with in realistic settings.

Linkages with operational health care programs will yield opportunities to include a variety of learning experiences in prevention, including participating in, planning, implementing, and evaluating preventive programs; developing relationships with consumers who are participants in health care programs; participating in medical practices in which prevention is regarded as an integral part of medical care; becoming part of efforts to influence agency or institutional policy with respect to prevention; working with community practitioners in their efforts to implement preventive programs; and so forth. These linkages can be seen in the context of developing competency-based approaches to educational and training programs for prevention (see Recommendations above).

Recommendations

1. That health sciences centers develop institution-wide approaches to planning, implementing, and managing education and training for prevention. That a preventive educational resource group be identified in each health sciences center as the major source of assistance in developing preventive content for curricula for each of the health professional programs and as the major focus in each center for research and advanced education relating to prevention. (Where appropriate, regional preventive educational resource groups could be set up.) That federal support can be provided for such institutionally planned and coordinated systems for education and training for prevention.

2. That educational and training programs for prevention develop close working relationships with operational health service agencies, institutions, and programs in which students and faculty can learn how to

cope with the major social, political, financial, administrative, and technical problems of prevention. That federal and other funding of educational and training programs for prevention take into account the educational importance of these operational settings.

3. That federal and other funding provide for the establishment of a small number of demonstration centers that incorporate the above mentioned concepts of (1) an institution-wide approach to planning and implementing educational programs for prevention, and (2) relationships with operational health service programs that will provide field settings for education and training for prevention.

Development and Dissemination of the Knowledge Base Necessary to Support Effective Education for Prevention

Proposition. An effective national effort directed toward prevention will depend heavily on the knowledge base developed through basic research and field studies. The ultimate usefulness of this knowledge depends, in turn, on its dissemination among health personnel through education and training. The existing knowledge base must be strengthened through the continued encouragement and support of research on prevention-related problems both by major educational and research institutions and by funding sources. Indeed, it would be the height of folly to mount a national preventive effort without ensuring a solid base of research and teacher training.

Substantiation. Splendid examples can be given of how research can contribute to the knowledge base for prevention and, subsequently, to its dissemination. The development of vaccines for polio and measles are two that come immediately to mind, and the control of viral hepatitis may be next in the line of serious diseases to be controlled by immunizing methods. What should not be overlooked is the wide range of disciplines that are essential in establishing such advances in preventive technology: a vaccine is developed by basic biomedical scientists working in interdisciplinary teams; its field testing is done by other teams—epidemiologists, biostatisticians, public health physicians and nurses; its incorporation into practice and evaluation are carried out first by teaching its use to health personnel and then by promotion, implementation, and follow-up studies by health care planners and administrators, clinicians, health educators, social scientists, and so forth.

Further examples come from the field of industrial health, where some discoveries are classic, such as the silicosis among rock and coal miners and lead poisoning among battery workers. Other problems are

71

currently generating great concern, such as the effects of asbestos and polyvinylpyrrolidine on people working with those materials. Here again, a combination of scientists from basic biomedical disciplines, clinical medicine, industrial health, epidemiology, and biostatistics, health care planners and administrators, and health educators interweave their efforts in identifying hazards to health and in developing practical, cost-effective efforts to protect workers and the public from exposure to them.

Of course, some of the most intractable preventable problems are based on human behavior, and a substantial proportion of future research efforts must focus on more effective ways of influencing health-related human behavior.

A key step in this process is the incorporation of these preventive concepts and skills into educational programs for various health personnel, and a key resource group for this purpose is specialists in the several fields of preventive medicine. Thus there need to be research and teacher-training programs for preventive medicine specialists as a critical component of prevention-oriented training institutions.

Regrettably, the agencies responsible for funding research in this country do not currently place a high priority on prevention-related problems, certainly not relative to the cost of providing medical care for those conditions after they have occurred. Even when research funds are available, support for training researchers and teachers is not. Research training grants have been very limited in recent years, and currently are nearly completely unavailable due to the President's decision to ask Congress to rescind monies already appropriated for these purposes. Thus, even the current research establishment is threatened, to say nothing of the research and training that would be needed on a much larger scale in order to provide the wider (and ever-widening) base required for a national approach to prevention.

Recommendations

1. That the Fogarty International Center and the American College of Preventive Medicine convene a working group to establish defensible priorities for recommendation to the federal government for expansion of support for research training programs in prevention-related basic science, clinical, public health and behavioral science disciplines.

2. That special emphasis be given in federal and other funding for research and teacher-training programs for specialists in preventive medicine as a critical component of prevention-oriented training programs for all health personnel.

72

Development of Educational and Training Continuums Corresponding to Planned Steps in Professional Development

Proposition. Education and training programs are usually discontinuous, with career dead-ends, lack of progressive programs that might provide continuity in educational development, and limited opportunity for mid-career changes. In addition, there is a shortage of informal, nondegree, noncourse study programs that are needed by professionals who want to improve their competence while remaining on the job. Thus, there is a need for educational and training continuums that correspond to planned steps of professional development, including mid-career changes.

Substantiation. The recent introduction at the state level of requirements for relicensure and recertification and the inclusion of similar concepts in national legislative proposals have laid bare serious deficiencies across the country in arrangements for continuing education. Career-long education for health professionals must be addressed in ways that systematically take into account the need for an educational continuum rather than a discontinuous and unplanned patchwork of programs. National and local governments, professional societies, and educational institutions need to be involved in this effort continuously and in concert, rather than sporadically and without coordination.

Much is said rhetorically about the importance of lifelong learning, but the capability for self-education needs to be supported by appropriate educational opportunities and by communications about newly legislated requirements, new manpower needs and opportunities, and new areas of technological innovation. Learning can be greatly enhanced by carefully planned programs on a lifelong basis as well as in the more structured settings of basic degree programs.

Since most of the manpower that would initially be involved in any national program for prevention would have already received their basic professional training, it is clear that the development of a national policy on prevention would necessitate providing the existing manpower pool with supplemental educational programs geared to their current responsibilities; the smaller group that wishes to make career changes would also require educational mechanisms that would cause a minimum of personal professional disruption.

Recommendations

1. That the health professions, through their professional societies and educational institutions, develop continuing education programs with preventive content, including:

a. Alternative long-range plans to fit a variety of professional needs, among them means for professional upgrading (including programs leading to certification and recertification and other kinds of "refresher" and "self-improvement" programs as well) and for offering basic degree requirements for persons wishing to extend their formal education—without necessarily requiring full-time academic work;

b. Appropriate educational materials, such as handbooks that delineate the specific competencies expected of various professional groups practicing in the field of prevention, self-instructional syllabi, and self-assessment examinations;

c. Regional "systems" of continuing education that will provide a basis not only for making coordinated use of regional resources, but also for meeting regional health manpower needs and certification requirements.

2. That federal and local governments, foundations, and educational institutions identify continuing education for prevention as an essential component of any national health manpower development strategy; that funding be made available for professional societies and educational institutions to develop continuing education programs; and that funding be made available to develop regional systems of continuing education.

The Relationship of Manpower Needs for Prevention to Education and Training Requirements

Proposition. Given both the costs and importance of health manpower, it is imperative that national and regional planning for manpower education and training proceed on a rational quantitative basis. Unfortunately, the data base needed to support such rational planning is seriously inadequate. It is essential, therefore, that prompt attention be given to improving the data system needed for health manpower planning. At the same time, there is sufficient evidence of current and prospective shortages in some manpower areas necessary to launching a national preventive effort to justify taking immediate steps to increase the education and training capacity for these categories.

Substantiation. While the need for a data system to support health manpower policy making is obvious, the inadequacies of the current data base with respect to prevention must be stressed: It is difficult to establish which occupational categories are mainly concerned with prevention, and even where specialty categories exist (as in board-certified specialists in preventive medicine), reliable supply data on numbers, employment, etc., are lacking. There is incomplete information on the preventive content both of basic professional educational programs and of the specialist programs for prevention. There is essentially no information about the present level of knowledge and skills needed for prevention among the current supply of health workers. Explicit norms are lacking for appropriate staffing patterns that could serve as a basis for projecting future requirements for manpower primarily concerned with prevention.

Health manpower is by far the most rapidly increasing major segment of the national labor force, growing during the 1965–1971 period alone by more than 60 percent, or 30 times the population growth rate and 15 times the rate of growth of the civilian labor force. With the manpower component accounting for well over one-half of the cost of health care, it is clearly in the government's interest to take prompt action to improve the quality and coverage of the data system required for manpower planning. The first priority should be given to strengthening the data base for the major categories of manpower that account for the bulk of the health labor force. In addition, however, concurrent measures on a pilot basis should be taken to improve the planning capabilities for certain "key" manpower categories, such as those concerned with prevention, which, even though they are not large numerically, can have a disproportionately significant impact on the effectiveness of health services. Planning for these key categories is especially complicated by their relatively greater dependence on social policy decisions and corresponding lesser reflection of market values. Means should also be developed for monitoring, on a sampling basis, certain aspects of the curricula of the principal health professions so that over time correlates can be developed between training and job effectiveness. The development of a health manpower statistical system capable of micro-studies on selected manpower categories and on complex topics such as the relationships between training and subsequent occupational performance will have to proceed cautiously lest costs become excessive, and great reliance will need to be placed on sampling. Nevertheless, Task Force V believes current efforts in these areas must be greatly strengthened if preventive services are to realize their full potential within the health care system.

Even though the Task Force recognizes that fine tuning of supply to meet anticipated requirements must await adequate data, it believes that there is already sufficient evidence of a shortage in certain manpower categories crucial to a national preventive effort to justify taking vigorous action now to increase supply. The manpower categories of particular concern are epidemiologists and biostatisticians, health services planners and administrators, health education specialists, and specialists in the preventive aspects of medicine, dentistry, and nursing.

Recommendations

1. That the federal government take steps immediately to increase the training capacities in the specialties listed below by one-third, to be accomplished by 1980 at the latest, with further increases to await the results of more detailed studies of requirements.

   a. Epidemiologists and Biostatisticians. These two manpower categories would provide for specialists in the measurement of health status, the study of the distribution and determinants of disease, and the evaluation of the effects of health care systems and technologies.

   b. Specialists in the Preventive Aspects of Medicine, Dentistry, and Nursing. These manpower categories are needed most urgently to expand and strengthen the preventive components of basic training in these professions. Physician specialists in preventive medicine (the four subspecialties—general preventive medicine, public health, occupational medicine, and aerospace medicine) have critical roles in research and training in prevention across the full spectrum of health problems and health personnel.

   c. Health Services Planners and Administrators. These manpower categories will have a critical role in the design and administration of health care systems that seek to combine efficiently the provision of both preventive and curative services.

   d. Health Education Specialists. The shortfall in this category is extreme. These personnel can provide leadership in the development of educational methods and programs aimed at improved health care and health-related behavior.

2. That the Fogarty International Center convene a working group that would include those concerned about health manpower for prevention and appropriate federal governmental agencies (including the National Center for Health Statistics and the Bureau of Health Manpower Education of HEW) to develop recommendations to the Department of Health, Education, and Welfare for developing a Health Manpower Statistical System capable of generating both the ongoing data needed for health manpower planning as well as carrying out special studies of topics of priority concern. DHEW and Congress have both had under consideration the creation of such a system for the past several years, though it is the Task Force's understanding that to date no final decisions have been made regarding implementation. As regards the area of special concern to this Task Force, it is recommended that the following efforts be pursued:

   a. That methods be developed that would allow monitoring of the training output and supply characteristics of those numerically small but highly specialized manpower categories concerned with prevention;

b. That economical methods be developed for the collection of information on selected components of curriculum content, including prevention. Such information would be extremely useful for improving educational programming, but without careful standardization of the data to be collected and the use of sampling techniques, such information would be both costly to obtain and perhaps of marginal utility.

c. That pilot programs and comparative research be intensified on topics of high priority, including relationships between variations in manpower inputs as regards preventive services and the resultant outputs and costs; relative benefits and limitations of different modalities of manpower training; and the ways in which differences in credentialing practices can affect manpower utilization and cost; and

d. That empirical models be developed for different prototypical health services, which would facilitate the study of interactions between various health manpower categories as regards such dimensions as productivity, substitutability, cost, and effectiveness. Over time, the postulated interactions should be replaced with actual data. By allowing planners and educators to take into account simultaneously more than a single manpower category, these models could greatly improve manpower planning.

Appendix A: Tracers of Other Manpower Categories

Tracer 1: Nutrition Services Personnel

This tracer was prepared by J. Warren Perry, PH.D., with the very generous assistance of a special task force from the American Dietetic Association.

Nutrition is an integral part of total health care throughout life, and dieticians and nutritionists are the only professionally educated group whose primary concern is the application of nutritional science to health care. As such, they should be involved in the planning and execution of all:

1. comprehensive health care programs;
2. nutrition education programs for the public; and
3. nutrition components in the training programs of all groups involved in health care and education.

Role

The dietician collaborates with others in planning, executing, and evaluating contributions to comprehensive health care programs. There are components of nutritional care in the prevention, treatment, and control of health problems of individuals, families, groups, and communities. This care may be given in a variety of settings: hospitals, extended care facilities, home care, community agencies, health maintenance organizations, ambulatory day care centers, and schools. Dieticians and nutritionists also have responsibility in areas of nutrition education and planning for nutritional care services for health protection and promotion, nutritional diagnosis and treatment, and appropriate referral.

Using the three-dimensional Prevention Matrix described above in Part II, one could demonstrate with numerous examples how the nutrition professional can play a wide and varied role in preventive health care. The following outline, for instance, depicts the activities of the dietician and the nutritionist in the prevention of cardiovascular disease:

Activity	*Target*
Health protection (general and specialized):	
1. Investigate, develop, and assess educational programs	1. Community

based upon nutritional label-
ing of foods
2. Institute regulations to permit
modification of needed foods
(as has been done in the case
of milk and ice milks contain-
ing 2 percent fat)   2. Community

Health education and promotion:
1. Publicize risk factors and provide public education, including such matters as tips for
weight control   1. Individual, family,
community
2. Encourage attendance at
screening programs   2. Individual, family,
community

Early diagnosis and treatment:
1. Follow up families of patients
with demonstrated disease
and assess dietary intakes   1. Family
2. Promote dietary modifica-
tions to achieve and maintain
decreased saturated fats and
cholesterol   2. Individual, family
3. Carry out vigorous therapy
with the patient related to
hyperlipidemic diagnosis   3. Individual
4. Monitor long-term adherence
to diet   4. Individual, family

Functions

Responsibilities and functions of dieticians and nutritionists in
health care settings that are adequately performed are:
1. Primary prevention (environmental protection, disease prevention, and health maintenance):
   a. assessment of food practices and nutritional status;
   b. referral;
   c. data input into patient information systems;
   d. individual diet counseling;
   e. group teaching;
   f. development and/or evaulation of nutrition teaching methods
   and materials;
   g. training and continuing education for dietetic supportive personnel;

    h. referral to and liaison with food assistance and other nutrition-related community programs; and

    i. consultation to group care facilities.

2. Secondary prevention in acute and intensive care:

    a. ongoing participation in health team planning, direct nutritional assessment, and counseling and evaluation;

    b. planning and/or supervision of appropriate group food services;

    c. dietetic information input in health team staff conferences; and

    d. initial and follow-up counseling in normal and therapeutic nutrition.

3. Secondary prevention in restorative and extended care:

    a. assistance in adjusting home environment to permit maximum independent functioning in activities in and out of the home; and

    b. liaison with noncontact services or programs helpful in carrying out the nutritional care plan.

Obstacles to Practice

The following deterrents in the health care system and professional education programs cause nutritionists and dieticians to *have difficulty in optimally carrying out their responsibilities*:

1. Recognition of the fact that nutritional care is basic to health care is absent.

2. Adequate funding for nutrition services in preventive care is not available.

3. Recognition of the need for ongoing support for research in the basic science of nutrition and in systems of nutritional care delivery is lacking.

4. Evaluation of applied nutrition programs for justification of continuation, expansion, or deletion is lacking. Government programs for supplying food to various target populations, such as food stamps, are commendable, but there should be reassessment and strengthening of *educational component* to achieve maximum benefit to health. For example, information on food safety and the nutrient adequacy of products is not always made available.

5. Preparation and continuing education in nutrition is not included in the curricula for medical, dental, and other professional health care personnel, thus preventing an interdisciplinary team approach to nutritional problems.

6. In part due to number 5, above, the potential for an expanded role of the dietician as a physician extender in planning and implementing

continuing care in settings outside acute care facilities has not been taken advantage of.

7. Diet counseling, initial and continuing, is not a reimbursable service in health insurance plans.

8. Nutritional status indices and dietary history and assessment are not always included in routine screening of patients. Even when such indices are included, referral to a nutrition professional does not always take place, in part, doubtless, because of number 7, above.

Recommendations

In order to plan and conduct optimal nutritional care programs with an emphasis on prevention, there is a need for change both in the health care *system* at large (policy, structure, and financing) and in the *education* the nutrition professional receives.

System changes. There is a need in the United States for a *national nutrition policy* that will ensure an available food supply; provide an adequate diet for all people at reasonable cost; disseminate information to the public relative to food and nutrition and its relationship to health status; and coordinate agricultural and nutrition policies. In addition, *structural changes* are needed in order to develop a system of coordinated nutrition programs, including the following:

1. adequate, wholesome food service;
2. nutrition education;
3. nutrition counseling for individual health problems;
4. linkages among all community health services and community nutrition programs;
5. research to provide knowledge in areas in which food and nutrition information is inadequate;
6. monitoring, surveillance, and periodic reporting on the prevalence of specific food and nutrition problems;
7. assessment and evaluation of preventive and remedial measures; and
8. program development that reflects findings of research, surveillance, and evaluation.

In order for these goals to be achieved, however, there will have to be *changes in the financing of nutritional care.* Such care, including nutritional counseling and nutrition education, should be identified and funded in all food assistance and health care programs. Programs for establishing and monitoring nutritional quality will require adequately prepared personnel and evaluation mechanisms to determine cost-effectiveness.

Educational needs. The following educational changes will have to be implemented in programs for training nutrition professionals in order to permit dieticians and nutritionists to provide optimal preventive services:

1. Nutrition education for the professional (and, indeed, for the public as well) must be related to the other health sciences; academic preparation for the nutrition-related professions should therefore be interdisciplinary with educational programs for other health professionals.

2. Centers of excellence for food and nutrition research and for the diagnosis and treatment of nutritional health problems should be developed.

3. Training of nutrition personnel should include experiences in both clinical and preventive health service settings (acute care, remedial care, and preventive care sites).

4. Educational programs should encompass the development of techniques in evaluation, including knowledge of the appropriate input of patient information into data systems.

5. Education and training for dietitians and nutritionists must include techniques in the management of people and resources.

6. Continuing education, both formal and informal, should be provided to assist the practitioner of nutrition services to maintain his or her competency in delivering care.

Manpower Considerations

This section of the tracer was written by Thomas L. Hall, M.D.

Educational requirements. Usual educational requirements for nutrition and dietetics personnel include a high school diploma and either a Bachelor of Science degree plus a one-year dietetic internship or a coordinated four-year B.S. program with specialization in nutrition. Personnel wishing to specialize in the community or large institutional aspects of this field may take a master's program, while those interested in research or teaching positions often go on to obtain a doctoral degree.

Supply. According to census data, the number of nutritionists and dieticians increased from 22,000 in 1950 to 41,000 in 1970, these figures giving an average annual rate of increase of 3.2 percent. If this rate is extrapolated to 1975, the number of nutritionists and dieticians employed would be about 48,000. Census data include persons with a wide variety of educational and occupational backgrounds, however, and the interest of this report is on those most directly concerned with preventive medicine. Other sources of supply estimates include the Institute of Food Technologists (12,392 members on April 1, 1974), the American School

82

Foodservice Association (54,178 members on March 11, 1975), and the American Dietetic Association (25,631 members on November 25, 1975). Undoubtedly there is significant overlap in these three associations, and for the most part those registered in the first two are of limited relevance to the concern of this report. The occupational breakdown of the ADA membership, given below, probably represents a closer approximation of those of primary concern.

Place of Employment

Hospital	10,477
Health care facility	1,751
College or university	1,958
Commercial or industrial	480
Government agency	594
School	1,028
Public health agency	840
Self-employed	647
More than one place	978
Outside of dietetics	447
Other	1,266

Major Responsibility

Teaching	2,237
Foodservice	1,306
Clinic therapeutic nutrition	4,984
General	2,916
Research	442
Management	3,032
Public health	795
Consultant	3,106
Other	1,624

Not listed in the above totals are some 5,165 inactive members or those for whom no occupational data are available. Of the nine categories listed, three (teaching, clinic therapeutic nutrition, and public health), accounting for 8,016 members, probably include those with the closest relation to preventive services.

Lastly, an estimate derived in 1973 placed the number of employed public health nutritionists with a graduate degree at between 1,000 and 1,200 during the early 1970s, a figure supported by the number of persons receiving a master's degree in this field (about 1,200 from 1946 through 1970).[1]

Proposed standards and projected manpower requirements. Various standards have been proposed for nutrition/dietetic personnel working in public health and preventive medicine capacities. The standards listed below may not be entirely mutually exclusive.

1. The Association of State and Territorial Nutrition Directors recommended in June 1974 to the Senate Select Committee on Nutrition and Human Needs a standard of one public health nutritionist per 50,000 population, along with sufficient supportive personnel. This would mean a 1980 requirement of almost 4,600 nutritionists and, although this standard did not specify the proposed level of training, it seems logical to assume that at least 50 percent (2,300+) should have advanced education in nutrition and public health.

2. State health departments with active nutrition programs are projecting current minimum needs at one nutritionist per 100,000 population, but for the most part their budgeted positions are coming nowhere near this standard. Florida, probably the best staffed, has 62 positions (about 40 in local health departments and 20 in state positions as supervisors, regional consultants, and special project personnel), or one per 125,000. Approximately two-thirds hold master's degrees, with the rest being registered dieticians, most with some baccalaureate training in community nutrition. The staffing rationale in Florida is one nutritionist for every ten public health nurses, or 1,000 hours of nutrition service per 50,000 population. In 1974, New York projected needs on the basis of one nutritionist for jurisdictions of 100,000 two for 500,000, and one for each additional 500,000 population.

3. The Health Insurance Plan of Greater New York (HIP), the prepaid health plan that has the most experience in offering nutrition services, contracts for one nutrition worker for every 20,000 enrollees. They utilize dieticians and persons with baccalaureate degrees in food and nutrition under the supervision of a public health nutritionist at a ratio of five to one. Applying this standard nationally in 1980 under the assumption of health care provided through an HMO-type system would result in a requirement of 11,400 nutrition workers, of whom about 1,900 would be public health nutritionists. [Actually, HIP is not strictly speaking an HMO (a couple of services that are mandated for an HMO are absent from the HIP benefit package). For our purposes here, however, it can be considered an HMO model.]

4. An ad hoc Task Force on Professional Health Manpower for Community Health Programs at the University of North Carolina estimated that based on the aggregation of proposed standards for public health nutritionists with master's- and doctoral-level training for a number of different work situations would result in requirements to for 1,600 persons in 1975, as against an estimated supply of 1,400 in the same year. The 1980 requirements and supply projections were 2,600 and 1,800, respectively.

5. In 1972 the Study Commission on Dietetics projected the need for professional dieticians and nutritionists by 1980 at 38,500, or approximately one professional per 5,900 population. The distribution according to functional area is: clinic practice, 25,000; food service management, 7,500; teaching, 1,500; commercial, 2,000; consumer health education and communication, 500; other, 1,000. If it is assumed that at a minimum the teaching, consumer health education, and one-half of the research category require postgraduate specialty training, this would mean a requirement of 2,500+ in 1980 with master's- and doctoral-level training.

The above standards are summarized below and applied to a projected 1980 population of 228 million.

Total requirements for professional *nutritionists and dieticians:*	38,500

Requirements for personnel with postbaccalaureate degrees, according to:

1. Association of State and Territorial Nutrition Directors	2,300+
2. State health departments (for state-level activities only)	2,300
3. University of North Carolina Task Force	2,600
4. Nationwide HMO system, based on HIP experience	1,900
5. Study Commission on Dietetics	2,500+

No information is available to indicate the extent to which the provision of nutrition services through a nationwide HMO system would reduce the requirements for nutrition personnel in governmental programs, though perhaps a safe assumption would be no more than a 50 percent overlap, i.e., that the implementation of a nationwide HMO system that provided nutrition services at the same level as HIP could reduce state and local governmental requirements by up to half, which would result in a national requirement of around 3,000 personnel with graduate degrees in 1980.

Projected balance between supply and requirements. The Task Force on Professional Health Manpower at the University of North Carolina estimated the number of employed persons with graduate degrees in public health nutrition at 1,000 in 1970 and projected a supply of 1,400 in 1975 and 1,800 in 1980. This assumes approximately 110 new graduates per year from existing programs. During the recent past, approximately 1,500 persons have graduated from baccalaureate nutrition programs annually and this number is expected to rise to 2,500 per year during the near future.[2] The training capacity of existing advanced degree programs could be expanded significantly with additional traineeships and the development of additional field training sites for public health and prevention activities. Even after taking into account a projected annual attrition rate of 3 percent for existing graduates and 2 percent for new graduates, the production of baccalaureate-level nutritionists and dieticians would seem adequate to meet probable requirements. However, the gap between the projected supply of and potential requirements for persons with advanced degrees could almost reach 1,000 in 1980 even without the full implementation of a nationwide HMO delivery system, which would be quite unlikely. Once such a system were implemented, the gap could increase far upwards of an additional 500.

When projecting a manpower shortfall it is important to consider whether a decision to increase supply would be matched by a comparable increase in job openings. At the present time, baccalaureate-level graduates are finding jobs in sick-care settings. Although there is no evidence of unemployment among graduates with advanced degrees, job opportunities in preventive medicine and public health settings are limited, due to the limited appreciation of the merits of utilizing nutrition personnel on health care teams. Moreover, in such jobs as are available, there is suggestive evidence that nutrition personnel are not being fully utilized in the preventive roles for which they were trained. For these reasons it would be important to match any efforts to increase the supply of nutrition personnel with specialty training in public health and preventive services with comparable efforts to increase job opportunities for the new graduates and improve the effectiveness of their utilization.

References

[1] Task Force on Professional Health Manpower for Community Health Programs (Thomas H. Hall, coordinator), *Professional Health Manpower for Community Health Programs,*

1973, Chapel Hill, N.C.: University of North Carolina, School of Public Health, Department of Health Administration, 1973, p. 92.

[2]John S. Millis, *The Profession of Dietetics: The Report of the Study Commission,* Chicago: American Dietetics Association. 1972, p. 53.

Tracer 2: General Dentistry Practitioner

This tracer was prepared by Rudolph E. Micik, M.S., D.D.S.

Introductory Remarks

Traditionally, the dental curriculum has provided the student with a comprehensive biomedical background and yet directed the graduate toward an almost total isolation from the general health care system. While an intensive basic science curriculum is presented to dental students, this training is not usually supported by any meaningful clinical medical experience. As a result, the dentist has tended to practice as a provider of treatment for specific dental and oral diseases, essentially segregated from other members of a health care team.

Recently, however, there have been a number of significant efforts within the dental profession and in schools of dentistry to stress the total health concept of care delivery. These developments are related to factors such as a renewed emphasis on prevention in dentistry, a greater delegation of tasks to auxiliaries, an increased awareness of dental disease on a community basis, and efforts to enhance the position of the generalist as a coordinator of health care.

The preventive dentistry model has sensitized many dentists to the significance of health maintenance through effective screening and diagnosis, preventive procedures, short- and long-term patient evaluation, and patient and public health education. Model programs are being initiated to broaden the dentist's undergraduate training in the area of diagnostic screening for medical problems and in the primary management of medical illness. Similar efforts are being considered for practicing dentists through graduate and continuing education courses. Thus it is expected that the general dental practitioner will become an important participant in the nation's total health manpower pool, particularly in the area of health protection.

Role

The preventive services rendered by the general dentist can be described in terms of the target and function axes of the Prevention Matrix in Part II above. Although not all dentists in fact routinely provide every service that will be mentioned here (a similar disclaimer could be made for all of the other health professionals for which tracer analyses have been included in this report), their education and training does qualify them for these activities.

Target: The Individual

I. Health Protection. The dentist:

A. Identifies the following factors that affect the onset and progression of oral and certain systemic diseases in the patient:

1. physical factors, including conditions apparent from patient's personal, medical, and dental history; the patient's general health status; local gingival irritants (plaque, calculus, restoration overhangs and contours, appliances); other soft tissue irritants (mechanical, chemical, thermal); and oral conditions that help determine the patient's caries potential (bacterial concentrations and activity, saliva flow and consistency, alignment relationship of the teeth, etc.);

2. psychological factors, including conditions such as anxiety and stress;

3. behavioral factors, including skill and frequency in plaque removal and patient's dietary practices, smoking habits, and drug intake;

4. educational factors, especially patient's ability to grasp oral health concepts; and

5. social and attitudinal factors, i.e., patient's attitude toward dental health and retention of natural dentition;

B. Provides the following preventive dental services to the patient:

1. prophylaxis (scaling and polishing, root planing);

2. application of preventive agents and devices (topical fluorides, night guards and mouth protectors, etc.);

3. prescription of preventive agents (e.g., fluoride dentifrices and beneficial nutritional elements);

4. removal of tissue irritants; and

5. maintenance of space and arch integrity;

C. Evaluates changes in patient's oral health status as a result of preventive services:

1. determines clinical changes;

2. assesses effects of proficiency and frequency of plaque removal, elimination of harmful oral habits, diet control, attitudes toward obtaining care, and self-screening skills; and

D. Refers patient for medical services when need is apparent.

II. Health Education. The dentist provides education on dental and medical preventive practices to develop patient's understanding of the needs for eliminating irritants and harmful habits, obtaining good nutrition, removing plaque, and obtaining prescribed professional care.

III. Early Diagnosis and Treatment. The dentist:

A. Identifies the presence and severity of oral diseases, particularly periodontal disease, dental caries, tooth and arch malalignment, and oral cancer;

B. Performs screening for potential medical problems, including:

1. taking and interpreting a brief medical history; and

2. conducting a head and neck examination, concentrating on the oral cavity, tonsillar area, and posterior pharynx;

C. Selects the appropriate care route for the patient:

1. refers patients with medical illnesses;

2. treats oral diseases;

3. refers patients with oral conditions requiring specialists;

4. maintains oral care for patient on a longitudinal basis (health maintenance).

Target: The Family

I. Health Protection. The dentist:

A. Obtains data on immediate family from patient (ages and medical and dental history); and

B. Prescribes preventive agents where indicated (e.g., systemic and topical fluorides).

II. Health Education. The dentist

A. Informs parent of potential oral health problems in infants and young children, including bottle-feeding problems and dietary factors;

B. Informs family member of potential oral health problems in the aged; and

C. Provides education on oral hygiene and nutrition for the family.

III. Early Diagnosis and Treatment. The dentist examines all family members as a unit where possible, noting family-associated factors affecting dental health and initiating intrafamily support for preventive measures.

Target: The Community

I. Health Protection and Education. The dentist

A. Promotes interest in community preventive dentistry programs (e.g., fluoridation of public water supply, preventive dentistry programs in schools, and public information programs) among local officials, institutions, agencies, and organizations; and

B. Serves as dental resource person for community dentistry programs.

Conclusions

General dentists could play a key role in preventive medicine. Many patients visit dentists on a regular basis, at which time certain systemic diseases, in addition to dental problems, could be detected at an early stage. The typical dental operatory already is, or easily can be, equipped to perform more thorough head and neck examinations and diagnostic procedures for certain high-risk conditions such as high blood pressure and diabetes. While, obviously, this would not substitute for a thorough periodic medical examination, it would nonetheless reach some people who would not otherwise receive any diagnostic treatment.

The major requirements for the maximum utilization of dental practitioners for such screening are: (1) some clinical training for medical procedures, (2) education for other professionals and the public on the expanded roles for dentists, and (3) mechanisms for enhanced interaction between dentists and other members of the health care team.

Manpower Considerations

This part of the tracer was written by Thomas L. Hall, M.D.

Increased interest in preventive dentistry in recent years has resulted in greater emphasis on this aspect of dental care in most dental schools in the United States. Increasingly, dental school curricula have stressed the importance of health maintenance through effective screening and diagnosis, preventive procedures, short- and long-term patient evaluation, and patient and public health education. Model programs have been initiated to broaden the dentist's undergraduate training in the area of diagnostic screening for medical problems and in the primary management of medical illness, while similar efforts are being considered for practicing dentists through graduate and continuing education courses. Nevertheless, preventive dentistry still receives relatively little emphasis in the total dental curriculum. It has been estimated that only 4 to 5 percent of the general dental education is focused on preventive care.[1]

One specialty that does focus primarily on the preventive aspects of dental care is public health dentistry. Public health dentists work at the federal, state, and local levels in the planning, implementation, management, and evaluation of dental health programs. They also participate as faculty and researchers in departments of community dentistry in dental schools and in schools of public health.

Present Educational Requirements. The educational requirements for general dentists are two to four years of college and four years of dental school. For those going on into public health dentistry, particularly those not involved in the direct provision of dental care, master's-level training

90

in public health dentistry and/or health administration is normally required. Most senior administrative and supervisory positions at federal, state, and local levels require a master's degree, as do many positions in dental schools and schools of public health.

Supply.   In 1970 there were approximately 102,000 active dentists in the United States, including about 7,000 federal dentists employed by the Armed Forces.[2] There was an approximate 30 percent increase in the number of active dentists between 1950 and 1970. Despite this increase during the 1950s and 1960s, there was a slight decline in the ratio of active dentists to total population from 51.5 per 100,000 population in 1950 to approximately 50 per 100,000 at the present time.

An ad hoc Task Force on Professional Health Manpower for Community Health Programs at the University of North Carolina estimated a supply of approximately 450 public health dentists in the United States in 1975. This figure was based on an estimate of 300 public health dentists in 1970 with approximately 30 graduates annually in the field during the 1970s. These estimates must be treated with caution, however, since they were not based on actual employment data, but rather on the number of degrees awarded.

Projected Supply.   As with most other health professions, the future supply of dentists largely reflects the growth of enrollments in professional schools. From 1953 to 1964, the number of graduates from U.S. dental schools rose at an average annual rate of approximately 1.2 percent. From 1965 through 1971, however, it averaged 3.1 percent, in large part as a result of federal support through basic improvement and special project grants and through the Health Professionals Educational Assistance Act. For their most recent series of supply projections as part of "Project SOAR" (Supply, Output, and Requirements), the Department of Health, Education, and Welfare assumed that when the current legislation expired in fiscal year 1974, there would be no extension of federal inducements to increase enrollments. They thus assumed a leveling off of enrollments and graduates of dental schools at the level reached in 1978–1979.[3]

The basic DHEW projection indicates that there will be a total gross graduate input of 74,700 over the 1971–1985 period. At the same time, the supply of active dentists is projected to grow from 102,220 in 1970 to 126,170 in 1980 and to 140,950 in 1985. The ratio of active dentists to population is projected to rise sharply in the future to a level of approximately 56 dentists per 100,000 population in 1980 and 59 per 100,000 in 1985; this compares with a ratio of 50 per 100,000 in 1970.

The University of North Carolina Task Force on Community Health Manpower projected the supply of public health dentists to be approximately 550 in 1980.[4] This projection was based on the assumptions of a supply of 300 public health dentists in 1970, additions at the rate of 30 new graduates in public health dentistry per year, 1970–1980, and a 1 percent annual loss of both the 1970 supply and the new graduates during that period. If the same assumptions are used and simply extended to 1985, the projected supply of public health dentists in 1985 would be approximately 675.

Requirements. A standard for the number of dentists required with adequate training in preventive dentistry and medical diagnosis has not been established. There appears to be an assumption that virtually all dentists should have the requisite training in preventive care, either as part of their undergraduate curriculum or through continuing education and graduate programs.

The standards for public health dentists used by the UNC Task Force on Professional Health Manpower presumed that these specialists would be employed primarily in administrative, policymaking, planning, evaluation, and academic positions. Using a series of estimates of the requirements for such dentists in different levels of government, educational institutions, and private industry, the UNC Task Force proposed a standard of approximately one public health dentist per 400,000 population in 1980. Assuming a population of 240 million in the United States in 1985, the requirements for public health dentists would be approximately 600.

Projected balance between supply and requirements. Although it has been estimated that in general the supply of dentists in 1985 will be adequate to meet the requirements, it must be recognized that probably no more than half of these dentists will have the requisite training in preventive dentistry. Assuming that virtually all of the new graduates from 1975 to 1985 receive such training in preventive dentistry and medical diagnosis, somewhat over 50 percent of the projected 140,000 active dentists in 1985 would have received such training. It is more realistic to assume, however, not only that somewhat less than 100 percent of the new graduates will have received the appropriate training, but also that approximately 5,000 at present are adequately qualified and some additional dentists out of the present supply will obtain training through continuing and graduate education programs. Thus, it seems a reasonable target for 1985 for 50 percent of all active dentists to have received the appropriate training in preventive dentistry and medical diagnosis.

In terms of public health dentists, the projected supply for 1985 will more than adequately meet the requirements set forth by the UNC Task Force on Professional Health Manpower. Still, it must be emphasized

92

that the standards used for obtaining those requirements were rather arbitrarily set to match the present supply in 1970, and that a number of contingencies could intervene to change the need for dentists with training in public health.

References

[1] Personal communication with Dr. Chester Douglass of the University of North Carolina School of Dentistry and School of Public Health.

[2] U.S. Department of Health, Education, and Welfare, Public Health Service, HSMHA, National Center for Health Statistics, *Health Resources Statistics*, 1971, Washington, D.C.: Government Printing Office, 1971.

[3] U.S. Department of Health, Education, and Welfare, *The Supply of Health Manpower: 1970 Profiles and Projections to 1990*, DHEW Publication No. (HRA) 75-38, December 1974, p. 82.

[4] Task Force on Professional Health Manpower for Community Health Programs (Thomas L. Hall, coordinator), *Professional Health Manpower for Community Health Programs, 1973*, Chapel Hill, N.C.: University of North Carolina, School of Public Health, Department of Health Administration, 1973, p. 83.

Tracer 3: Certified Nurse-Midwife

This tracer topic was selected by Thelma Ingles, M.A., R.N., who feels that this particular area of nursing will be of increasing importance in health care. She points out that although the details of the tracer would differ, many of the principles derived from this analysis would apply equally well to other types of nurse-practitioners. Dorothea M. Lang, C.N.M., M.P.H., provided assistance in developing the tracer.

Introduction

This overview of the certified nurse-midwife (C.N.M.) is an example of a nonphysician professional's participation in preventive medicine. The scope and practice of midwifery has been well recognized around the world, where 80 percent of all babies born are delivered by nonphysicians. In the countries that have the lowest infant mortality rate, care by a midwife is the norm (1973 rate in Sweden, 9.9; Finland, 10.1; Netherlands, 11.5; Japan, 11.3).[1,2] Similarly, the increasing utilization of the certified nurse-midwife in the United States shows that this professional is contributing a favorable new dimension to the health team in preventive health care.

93

Role

Using the Prevention Matrix in Part II to identify the activities and targets of the certified nurse-midwife reveals that this professional is prepared by education and experience to carry primary responsibilities for health protection, health education, and early diagnosis and treatment of patients throughout the maternity cycle. In addition, she provides necessary support through education and guidance for families, and participates in community activities that relate to women's health and maternal and infant care.

As part of the professional team of a hospital or health service, the certified nurse-midwife functions in reproductive health maintenance of women and provides prenatal care, labor and delivery services, postpartum care, family planning, pre- and interconceptional health care, and related health education and counseling. Perinatal care, newborn screening, and family health counseling are also part of midwifery practice. Certified nurse-midwives practice in a framework of an organized regional or local health service with qualified medical direction.

Scope of Practice, Functions, and Responsibilities [3,4]

The certified nurse-midwife functions in various settings. She may be employed by a hospital, by a medical-center-affiliated maternal and child health service, by a community-based health station or center, or by an obstetrician/midwife group practice.

Midwifery practice encompasses the philosophy that each woman has the right to preventive and personalized health care, and the right to acquire health education in order to understand her own psychophysiologic functions as woman, mate, and mother. This means that along with quality physical care, the midwife also provides family-life education opportunities which will guide the woman and her family toward "self-preservation of health." In addition, the C.N.M. screens for and refers any medical or mental health problems to the appropriate medical specialist.

Preventive medicine as practiced by the certified nurse-midwife includes the awareness that childbearing is a family experience and encourages active involvement of family members in care. This family-centered preventive health management combined with individualized health education guides the consumer toward:
1. quality in the childbrith experience;
2. satisfaction in nurturing the newborn;
3. security, as desired, through personalized family planning; and
4. the ability to form rewarding family relationship within the cultural setting of one's choosing.

In an increasing number of urban and rural settings, the certified nurse-midwife provides complete reproductive health care for medically uncomplicated, low-risk patients. Mothers with obstetrical complications are co-managed with the OB/GYN specialist. The physician manages the medical problems, and the midwife manages the uncomplicated course of labor and spontaneous delivery. Preventive newborn care is managed by the midwife in consultation with the perinatologist, neonatologist, or pediatrician.

For patients desiring interconceptual care, the midwife provides family planning services, as desired and as medically suitable to the patient's needs. Personal hygiene information, family planning, and sex counseling are provided simultaneously. Routine breast examinations, Pap tests, lab tests, and simple gynecologic procedures are also performed by the midwife, as agreed upon by the obstetrician/midwife team and specified in written protocols (approved orders).

Midwives frequently provide preventive health care for teenagers. This appears to ease the adjustment of the teenager to unexpected pregnancy and motherhood (or family planning). This personalized non-"paternalistic" type of primary care as provided by the C.N.M. seems to be less threatening to the adolescent or young adult, who then more readily accepts additional medical care or the valuable counseling of the public health nurse, nutritionist, social worker, or other health team member.

Consumer acceptance of midwifery services are overwhelmingly positive.

In addition to providing primary care and health education for individual patients and their families, midwives also participate in the following community-based activities:

1. functions as a health advocate for the female patient (and her family) between community and hospital-based facilities;

2. plans and provides educational programs for parenting, including fetal growth and development, normal growth and health protection (hygiene; nutrition, including breast feeding; immunization schedule; safety methods and avoidance of hazards), and mental health needs, including family planning;

3. provides classes in sex education for school children;

4. provides individual and group counseling in hygiene and women's preventive health care measures, venereal disease prevention, sex education, contraception, infertility prevention, breast self-examination, gynecologic cancer screening, women's health needs during years of menstruation and menopause;

5. participates in community-based health screening endeavors for cancer and pregnancy;

6. participates actively in civic affairs that reflect on maternal and child health and family life.

Justification for the Utilization of Certified Nurse-Midwives to Further the Goals of Preventive Medicine

There is ample justification, from a preventive point of view, for increasing the use of certified nurse-midwives in obstetrical and family care. These professional midwives permit a more efficient and effective means of providing preventive medical services than the traditional methods and organizations offer, as the following points will document:

1. To provide optimally integrated services the responsibility for health protection and health education in maternity care should rest with the same health professionals who provide medical care. Midwifery care encompasses both.

2. There are indications that the use of professional midwives plays a role in the reduction of infant and maternal morbidity and mortality. In countries with maternal and infant morbidity and mortality rates superior to those in the United States, midwives are much more prevalent. This relationship has been substantiated by data from the United States as well. The following examples are only several among many that could be cited. While the data given here are incomplete, they suggest that C.N.M.s can make important contributions in a variety of settings.

A. *Kentucky's Midwifery Program of the Frontier Nursing Service (FNS).* Despite the high poverty level and minimal education of the population of the region served by the Frontier Nursing Service, the infant mortality and morbidity rates have been superior to those of the country as a whole. This is primarily attributed to the services provided by the midwives of FNS. There were no maternal deaths at the FNS since 1952.

Birthrate in Leslie County, Kentucky (FNS area):
   1953: 41 per 1000
   1973: 18 per 1000
Stillbirths in FNS area:
   1950–1970: fell from 16.5 to 10.1 per 1000 live births
Puerperal mortality rate:
   1925–1955
      FNS area: 9.1 per 10,000 live births
      USA: 34.0 per 10,000 live births
   1950–1970
      FNS area: 1.2 per 10,000 live births
      All Kentucky: 2.1 per 10,000 live births

B. *Madera County Midwifery Project, California.*[5] The ability of certified nurse-midwives to upgrade the quality of care to childbearing

96

women was well documented in a demonstration project in a rural hospital in the 1960s, with the following results:

1. Mothers were attended throughout labor.
2. The course of labor was observed more carefully with better recording.
3. Consultation was prompt and easily obtainable. Delivery by unprepared attendants was reduced.
4. Incidence of prematurity rate declined: 1959: 11.0 percent before midwifery project 1961: 6.4 percent during midwifery project
5. Neonatal deaths decreased strikingly: 1959: 23.9 per 1,000 live births before project; 1961: 10.3 per 1,000 live births during project.

C. *Presbyterian Hospital's Midwifery Program, New York City.*[6] In one study, over 100 pregnant teenagers between the ages of thirteen and eighteen were provided prenatal care by a midwife. All had many of the "typical" inner-city socioeconomic problems and were therefore considered to be in a high-risk category. The pregnancy outcome showed a remarkably low prematurity rate of 5.3 percent, as compared to New York City's overall rate of 9.2 percent. The mean newborn weight was excellent, a surprising 3200 gms. The teenagers averaged nine prenatal visits each, and all attended at least six young parents group education sessions.

In general, the large-scale use of midwives in every community would enhance and increase the scope of preventive health care for specific target groups such as female adolescents, women in their reproductive years, newborns and infants during the first year of life. Secondary benefits would also be realized by the increased health education and resultant well-being of the mother that will be influential in increasing the health standards for the whole family and future generations.

Discrepancies Between Current and Desired Practice

Difficulties encountered by certified nurse-midwives in effectively carrying out the responsibilities for which they were educated include not only many of the same system problmes that impede the practice of preventive care by other providers in other medical fields, but also the following:

1. Hospital administrators are reluctant to designate a budget for the employment of midwives, chiefly because professional midwifery is a comparatively new concept in American health care and administrators are therefore uncertain of how to determine staffing requirements utilizing C.N.M.s and how to cost-account midwives into their hospital's fiscal plans. There is also sometimes fear on the part of administrators who

97

have no experience in settings where nurse-midwives have been employed that midwives would not be well accepted by physicians and/or obstetrical nurses.

2. Although all but two states have enabling laws that permit professional midwifery services to be provided by the certified nurse-midwife, many states have not yet adjusted their laws and health codes so that C.N.M.s can fully function on the health team (e.g., although normal obstetrical/midwifery management requires the prescribing of simple medications, oxytocins, specific narcotics, and sedatives for analgesia during labor, the laws in many states have not been adapted to make certified nurse-midwives an exception to the rule that only licensed physicians and dentists may prescribe medications. In most countries midwives are assigned by law a circumscribed list of medications and narcotics from which they can select and prescribe as required for midwifery management.)[7]

3. Increasingly less, but nevertheless still occasionally, the certified nurse-midwife is confused by public with the self-appointed lay midwife. Lay midwives are not eligible for current state licensure anywhere in this country (with the single exception of a few "granny" lay midwives in the south). Nevertheless, "the word 'midwife' still makes some people think of a toothless crone boiling a teakettle of water in a shack somewhere in Kentucky, while the pregnant woman's husband quaffs corn liquor in the next room."[8] The last vestiges of this erroneous image need to be eradicated.

Implications for Changes in the Health Care System and Recommendations

It is not likely that professional midwives will be able to function up to their capacity and training in all areas of the country unless at least some of the following major changes occur:

1. The first of the above-mentioned obstacles to the effective performance of midwives, the reluctance of hospital administrators to hire and budget for them, must be removed. Demonstration funds should be made available and national health policies should encourage employment of midwives by health care facilities. Acceptance of the professional midwife by consumers has been overwhelmingly positive. Acceptance by the health professionals will be enhanced by repeated exposure of the midwife to the health team. Government funding of midwifery and medical education should encourage a multidisciplinary approach to learning, with ample exposure for all students to preventive medicine and public health. The acceptance of C.N.M.s as essential members of primary care teams would be encouraged if part of the training for nurse-midwives and

other health professionals alike (physicians, administrators, etc.) occurred within a regional medical health care setting.

2. The years of education for a certified nurse-midwife are less than half the number of academic and training years required to educate an obstetrician. It therefore makes good sense just in terms of the rational use of resources to allocate more funds to midwifery education than are currently made available. Financial support should be given not only to expanding current midwifery programs, but also to increasing the number of such programs. (There are presently only eighteen in the United States, and there are currently at least fifty additional qualified applicants that each school must turn down every year due to the limited size of the programs.)

3. Educational programs should be encouraged to allow lateral mobility among health professionals in preventive medicine. This is possible because midwifery educational programs can exist in affiliation with a variety of university faculties—schools of public health, medical schools, schools of nursing, and schools of allied health sciences.

4. In order for clinical instructors in midwifery education programs to receive the necessary midwifery experience a patient-service setting prior to assuming teaching responsibilities, funding is needed to support midwives with master's degrees for a period of two years each.

5. Increasing numbers of college-educated women without a nursing education have also expressed interest in entering the profession of midwifery. Health sciences centers should investigate establishing a joint program for such candidates, perhaps leading to a combined R.N./C.N.M. degree.

6. Evaluation of midwifery care should be provided at the same time that all obstetric/gynecologic services are evaluated. Evaluations should be conducted by peer review including a team of physicians and midwives.

7. The problem cited in No. 2 in the list of obstacles to practice above, i.e., the existence of certain state laws and health codes that prohibit the C.N.M. from performing certain functions for which she is completely qualified and thoroughly trained, must be solved by emending those regulations.

8. In reference to No. 3 in the list of discrepancies between current and desired practice, additional public education is needed to inform the consumer (and some providers as well) of the existence of the professional midwife and of her capabilities and qualifications.

Manpower Considerations

This section of the tracer was prepared by Thomas L. Hall, M.D.

The more than one hundred midwifery services that exist in affiliation with obstetrical services of hospitals and medical centers throughout the country are a demonstration of the successful utilization of these nonphysician professionals to further the goals of preventive medicine.

The nurse-midwife is a registered nurse (R.N.) who has successfully completed one of two types of programs: (1) a course of study, usually 6 to 8 months in length—plus clinical experience—leading to a certificate in nurse-midwifery, or (2) advanced preparation and clinical experience in a college or university program, usually 12 to 24 months in length, leading to a master's degree and to a certificate in nurse-midwifery. The number of programs preparing nurse-midwives at the master's level has increased as the number of programs leading to just a certificate has decreased. Schools of nurse-midwifery are approved by the American College of Nurse-Midwives (ACNM), the national professional organization.

Approximately 85 nurse-midwives graduate each year from U.S. schools of nurse-midwifery. After graduation from a school of nurse-midwifery approved by the American College of Nurse-Midwives (621 members) or, in the case of the foreign-prepared graduate, written evidence that specified criteria established by the College have been met, the nurse-midwife is eligible to take the ACNM certification examination. Successful completion of the examination qualifies the nurse-midwife to use the title certified nurse-midwife (C.N.M.). To date, 800 persons have been certified.[9]

Supply. In 1973, there were an estimated 1,300 nurse-midwives in the United States, most of whom practice in the eastern part of the country.[10]

Requirements. Little information is available on the requirements for nurse-midwives in the United States. A brief search of the literature was made to determine if standards for requirements for nurse-midwives had been set for any of the European countries, but nothing definitive was found. A spokesman for the ACNM, however, indicated that currently every graduate of a nurse-midwifery program gets at least ten job offers from across the country, which would seem to indicate considerable demand for these professionals. The same source further estimated that at least three midwives could be effectively utilized as members of the obstetrical team in every hospital with a major OB/GYN service. Depending, of course, on how one defines "major OB/GYN service," that could mean a present requirement for as many as 7,000 hospital-based nurse-midwives alone.

References

[1] United Nations Office of Statistics, February 1975.

[2] International Federation of Gynecology and Obstetrics and the International Confederation of Midwives, *Maternity Care Around the World: An International Survey of Midwifery Practice and Training*, Elmsford, N.Y.: Pergamon Press, 1966

[3] *Functions, Standards, and Qualifications*, American College of Nurse-Midwives, 1000 Vermont Ave., N.W., Washington, D.C. 20005.

[4] American College of Obstetricians and Gynecologists (ACOG), the Nurses Association of the American College of Obstetricians and Gynecologists (NAACOG), and the American College of Nurse-Midwives (ACNM), *Joint Statement on Maternity Care*, February 1971. A *Supplement* statement is currently being developed by these professional organizations that will further enhance this nonphysician professional's function on regional health teams.

[5] B.S. Levy, F.S. Wilkinson, and W.M. Marine, "Reducing the Neonatal Mortality Rate with Nurse-Midwives," *American Journal of Obstetrics and Gynecology*, 109, no. 1 (January 1971).

[6] Mildred Abbott, "A Pregnant Approach to Teenage Antepartum Care" (to be published).

[7] *Survey of Legislation Pertaining to the Practice of Nurse-Midwifery*, American College of Nurse-Midwives, Washington, D.C.

[8] Judy Klemestrud, "Midwives Carry New Image into Hospital Delivery Room," *The New York Times*, Sept. 20, 1971.

[9] United States Department of Health, Education, and Welfare, Public Health Service, HRA, National Center for Health Statistics, *Health Resources Statistics*, 1974, Washington, D.C.: Government Printing Office, 1974, p. 193.

[10] *Ibid.*

Appendix B: Community-Oriented Roles to be Addressed in the Education of Primary Care Physicians

WILLIAM H. BARKER, M.D.

In addition to preparing primary care physicians to play a direct role in delivering personal preventive health services (as discussed in the Tracer of the Family Physician in Part II of this report and delineated in detail in the report of Task Force III), education for preventive/community medicine should ·prepare physicians to play certain important indirect roles in linking patient care with community-based preventive health services. ("Community-based preventive health services" in this context consist of the wide variety of public and voluntary agencies or organizations that have developed historically to meet those various disease control and health maintenance needs of communities and individuals which are not met through the traditional doctor-patient medical care model.)

The proposed community-oriented preventive roles for which practitioners should be educated are subsumed under the following two generic functions, both of which derive naturally from the doctor-patient medical care model:

1. *Referral* of individual patients to community agencies that provide supportive, rehabilitative, or other special personal services which physicians cannot readily provide in their practice setting. Such services might include Alcoholics Anonymous, occupational and physical rehabilitation, family planning, crippled children's programs, smoking and weight control programs, etc. The most effective way to prepare physicians for this role remains to be determined. Presumably a physician would need to have command of the following:

1. a body of knowledge regarding the availability and operating procedure of such community services;
2. evaluative skills for determining the effectiveness of a particular service;
3. management skills to facilitate communication with community service personnel regarding a patient's needs.

2. *Reporting* to designated community or institutional health authorities those patients presenting with preventable illnesses that might signify an ongoing but controllable community health hazard. Included among such reportable diseases are the officially notifiable communicable diseases, nosocomial infections, poisoning from hazards in the home or community environment (e.g., lead and carbon monoxide), occupationally acquired illness, etc. In addition, the practicing physician could contribute to the recognition and control of newly occurring preventable problems by reporting unusual clusters or patterns of illness seen in practice; this is particularly pertinent to the recognition of adverse effects of new drugs and medical devices.

Preparation of practising physicians for this epidemiologic surveillance role would include imparting to them the following:

1. a thorough understanding of the epidemiologic precepts of disease determinants (host, agent, and environment antecedents) and distribution (persons at risk);

2. an ability to routinely apply these epidemiologic precepts in recognizing patients whose illnesses have preventable antecedents and hence may have preventive implications for others at risk in the community;

3. a body of knowledge regarding those diseases known to have such community preventive implications.

4. a familiarity with the operations of community or institutional programs for controlling such diseases, particularly the notification aspect (including local, state, and federal communicable disease, environmental, and occupational health programs, etc.).

These community-oriented elements of physician training might best be provided through first-hand experience working with community-based services. This would require the establishment of educational affiliations between medical schools or primary care residency programs and various public and voluntary community agencies. According to a recent survey of teaching programs in departments of preventive/community medicine in United States medical schools that was conducted by the Association of Teachers of Preventive Medicine, the majority of schools provide minimal or no educational experience with such agencies. There is little available information on the current state of community-oriented training in primary care residency programs in the country.

The following selected references provide some of the conceptual and factual knowledge appropriate to teaching the community-oriented roles of the practicing physician.

References

W.H. Barker, ed., *Preventive/Community Medicine in the Education of Primary Care Physicians*. Proceedings of Association of Teachers of Preventive Medicine-Fogarty International Center Workshop (to be published).

A.S. Benenson, ed., *Control of Communicable Diseases in Man*. Washington D.C.: American Public Health Association, 1970.

J.B.M. Davies, *Preventive Medicine, Community Health and Social Services*. London: Balliere, Tindall, and Cassell Ltd., 1971.

R.L. Kane, ed., *The Challenges of Community Medicine*. New York: Springer Publishing Company, 1974.

S.L. Kark, *Epidemiology and Community Medicine*. New York: Appleton-Century-Crofts, 1974.

J.N. Morris, *Uses of Epidemiology*. Edinburgh: E. and S. Livingstone, 1970.

Appendix C: The American Board of Medical Specialties

Recommended Guidelines on Recertification for Specialty Boards

1. Recertification should assure, through periodic evaluations, the physician's continuing competence in his chosen area of specialty practice.

2. Recertification should encourage certified physicians to continue those educational activities essential to the maintenance of competence in their specialties.
3. It is the prerogative of individual boards to elect voluntary or mandatory recertification; however, a specialty board may not rescind initial certificates by recertification procedures unless a date of expiration was a condition of the original certification.
4. Similar intervals for recertification by the specialty boards are desirable; an appropriate interval appears to be six years but not more than ten.
5. Upon recertification, the listing of a specialist in the *Directory of Medical Specialists* will include the date of original certification and the dates of any recertifications.
6. Recertification may apply to any of the fields in which a specialty board grants certificates.
7. Member boards are encouraged to develop procedures for recertification that are most appropriate to the characteristics of their specialty practice. Evaluated participation in continuing education, oral or written cognitive examinations, skills and performance evaluations, practice audits and practice profiles are among the elements that should be considered and utilized as may be appropriate and with suitable emphasis or weighting.
8. Policies and procedures for recertification should be incorporated in the published requirements for certification provided by each specialty board.
9. In the light of rapid developments now taking place in examination and testing technics, Member Boards are also encouraged to review on a continuing basis the recertification procedures they may develop and adopt.
10. The design of recertification procedures requires close collaboration between specialty boards and their related specialty societies and other constituencies; however, the determination of policies and procedures affecting the recertification process is ultimately the responsibility of each primary or conjoint board.

Appendix D: Core Curriculum Materials in Preventive Medicine for Undergraduate Medical Education:

A Project Being Developed Jointly by the Association of Teachers of Preventive Medicine and Harvard's Center for Educational Development in Health

Achievement of a comprehensive preventive approach in medical practice depends on a complex of factors. One key component is the preparation of physicians in various specialties to apply preventive concepts effectively in their respective professional practices.

While it is clear that factors other than training play a role, such as incentives, patient receptivity, and community support at various levels, it is equally clear that physicians can act preventively only to the extent that their skills and knowledge enable them to, which means, in effect, that undergraduate medical education must become increasingly relevant to the demands of preventive practice. Medical students must have access—independently of their intended specialty—to effective preventive medicine instruction, if they are to be expected to function preventively in their practices.

In this context, an especially interesting project is that proposed jointly by the Association of Teachers of Preventive Medicine (ATPM) and the Harvard Center for Educational Development in Health (CEDH) for development of core curriculum materials in preventive medicine for use in undergraduate medical education.

The distinctive feature of the project is its provision for ensuring inputs from various medical specialty societies in the establishment of a competency-based curriculum. The instructional objectives will be derived from the systematic effort by teams of medical specialists and instructional technologists to define skills and knowledge required for effective preventive medical practice.

The resulting core curriculum instructional materials—to be field-tested to ensure their effectiveness—will be organized into modules for flexible, individualized administration. The modules will rely substantially on available instructional resources, and only those teaching materials will be developed that are found necessary to fill gaps.

The project envisions a series of phases encompassing curriculum design, materials development, field testing, and the planning of a dissemination system. Direction of project activities will be by a task force of ATPM and CEDH personnel, who will work closely with physicians representing various specialties to ensure that the curriculum objectives and materials reflect the needs of practicing physicians with respect to effective application of preventive medicine concepts.

In the critical first phase, a systematic curriculum design process developed by CEDH personnel will be used to define a competency-based curriculum in the form of behaviorally specified, systematically organized instructional objectives from which the instructional modules will be developed and tested in the subsequent phases. Teams of specialists will identify skills and knowledge required to apply preventive concepts. Their recommendations will then be submitted to representative samples of various medical specialties for verification.